Anshan Gold Standard Mini Atlas Series

Color Doppler

Satish K Bhargava
MD (Radiodiagnosis), MD (Radiotherapy)
DMRD, FICR, FIAMS, FCCP, FIMSA, FAMS
Professor and Head
Department of Radiology and Imaging
University College of Medical Sciences (Delhi University)
and associated GTB Hospital
Delhi, India

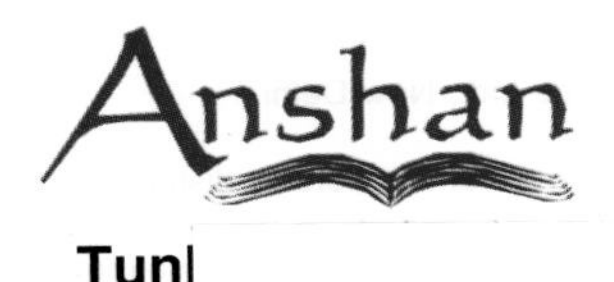

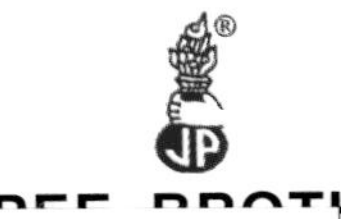

JAYPEE BROTHERS
Tunl
(P) LTD.

CONTRIBUTORS

Satish K Bhargava
Head, Dept of Radiology and Imaging
University College of Medical Sciences (Delhi University)
and associated GTB Hospital, Delhi, India

Rajul Rastogi
Ex-Resident, Dept of Radiology and Imaging
University College of Medical Sciences (Delhi University)
and associated GTB Hospital, Delhi 110095
At present, Yash Diagnostic Hospital and Research Center,
Civil Lines, Kanth Road, Moradabad, Uttar Pradesh, India

Sumeet Bhargava
Ex-Resident, Dept of Radiology and Imaging
University College of Medical Sciences (Delhi University)
and associated GTB Hospital, Delhi 110095
At present, Dewan Chandra Satya Pal Aggarwal Imaging
Center, 10-B, Kasturba Gandhi Marg, New Delhi India

Anurag Agarwal
Ex-Resident, Maulana Azad Medical College and
associated LNJP Hospital, New Delhi, India

PREFACE

The first edition of Anshan Gold Standard Mini Atlas Series—Color Doppler is being brought out on the demand of several students of Radiology, who want to have a quick review of Color Doppler Spectrum—Normal and Abnormal. This mini atlas includes brief account of most of the common lesions as well as common Doppler spectra. All are with illustrations.

The Mini Atlas Series is a vision and sincere effort of Shri Jitendar P Vij (CEO) of M/s Jaypee Brothers Medical Publishers (P) Ltd on the demands and expectations of a large number of readers all over the world. The staff of M/s Jaypee Brothers Medical Publishers (P) Ltd particularly Mr Tarun Duneja (Director-Publishing) and Samina Khan along with others are quite helpful and praiseworthy.

At last, valuable suggestion from the readers will be very useful to improve it further and will be greatly acknowledged.

Satish K Bhargava

CONTENTS

Chapter One

Basic Principles

DOPPLER INDICES

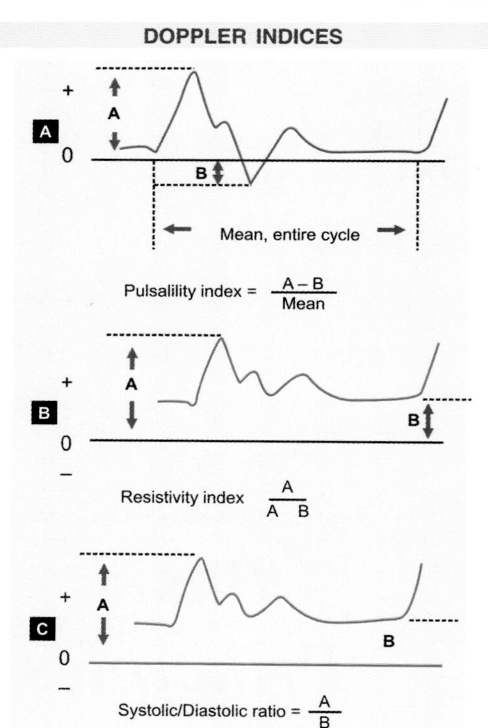

FIGURES 1.1A to C

(A) The pulsatility index or Gosling & King index (PSV-EDV/Mean Velocity), (B) The resistivity index or Pourcelot index (PSV-EDV/EDV), (C) The systolic/diastolic ratio or Stuart index (PSV/EDV)

These indices are independent of their beam angle and are therefore unaffected by imprecise angle data

NORMAL FLOW IN CENTRAL VEIN

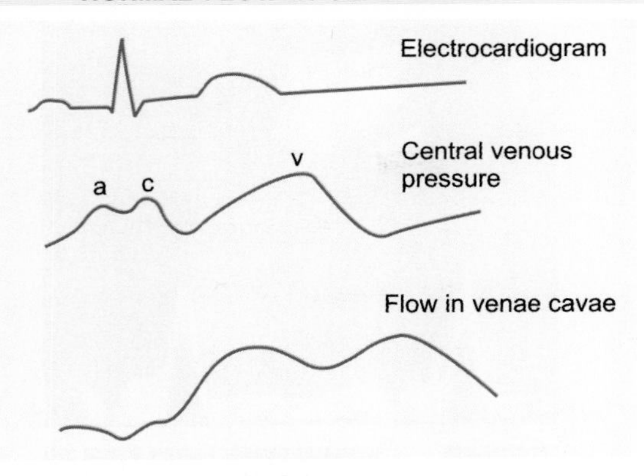

FIGURE 1.2

Schematic representation of normal changes in pressure and flow in the central veins associated with the cardiac cycle.

a = a wave is caused by atrial contraction against the closed atrioventricular valve

c = c wave is caused by bulging of the atrioventricular valves into the atrial cavity during isovolumetric ventricular contraction

v = v wave is caused by the rise in atrial pressure during filling of atria from peripheral veins during ventricular emptying

THE DOPPLER SPECTRUM DISPLAY

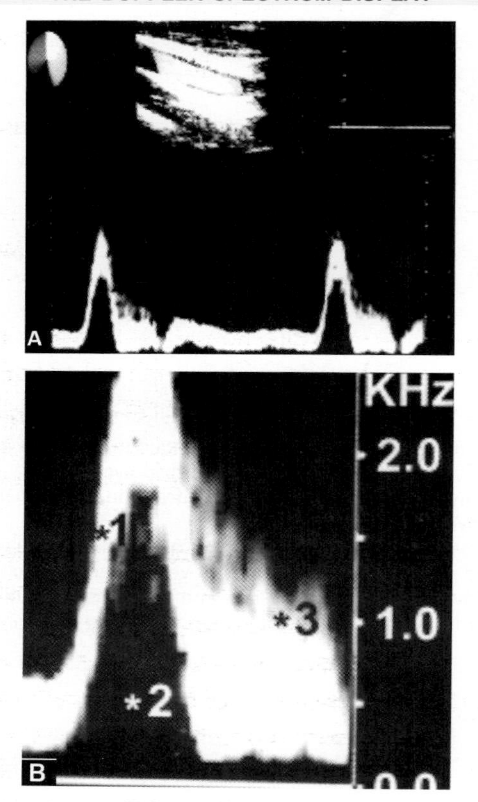

FIGURES 1.3A and B

The following information is presented on the display screen (A) entire display; (B) magnified Doppler spectrum

B-mode image: The image of the vessel, the sample volume and the Doppler line of sight are shown at the top of the display screen.

Time: It is represented on the horizontal (x) axis of the Doppler spectrum in divisions of a second.

Frequency shift and velocity: The Doppler frequency shift (kHz) and the velocity (cm/sec) are shown on the vertical (y-axis) scales of the spectrum.

Flow direction: The direction of flow is shown in relation to the spectrum baseline. For peripheral vascular work, flow away from the transducer is shown above the baseline, and flow towards the transducer is shown below the baseline. This relationship may be reversed by the operator.

The distribution of velocities within the sample volume is illustrated by the brightness of the spectral display (z-axis). To better understand the z-axis concept, examine the magnified spectrum shown in B and imagine that the spectral display is made up of tiny squares called pixels (for picture elements). You cannot see the pixels in this image, because they are purposely blurred together to smooth the picture. The pixels are there, however, and each corresponds to a specific moment in time and a specific frequency shift and velocity. The brightness of a pixel (z-axis) is proportionate to the number of blood cells causing that frequency shift at that specific point in time. In this example, the pixels at asterisk 1 are bright white, meaning that at that movement, a large number of blood cells have a velocity corresponding to a frequency shift of +1.5 kHz. The pixels at asterisk 2 are black, meaning that at that movement, no (or very few) blood cells have a velocity corresponding to a frequency shift of +0.5 kHz. The pixels at asterisk 3 are gray, meaning that at that a moderate number of blood cells have a velocity corresponding to a +0.5 kHz frequency shift at that moment.

PERIPHERAL RESISTANCE ON DOPPLER SPECTRA

Influence of the peripheral resistance on Doppler spectra recorded from the brachial artery (A, B) and internal carotid artery (C) in a healthy subject.

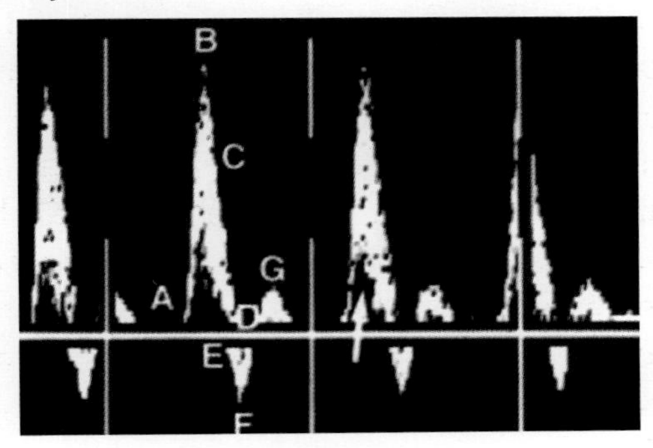

FIGURE 1.4A

Triphasic spectrum at rest. High peripheral vascular flow resistance (peripheral-artery pattern) with a sharp systolic velocity increase (A-B), a rapid drop in velocity in late systole (C-D), diastolic flow reversal (E-F), and late diastolic forward flow (G). Note the spectral window below the systolic peak (white arrow)

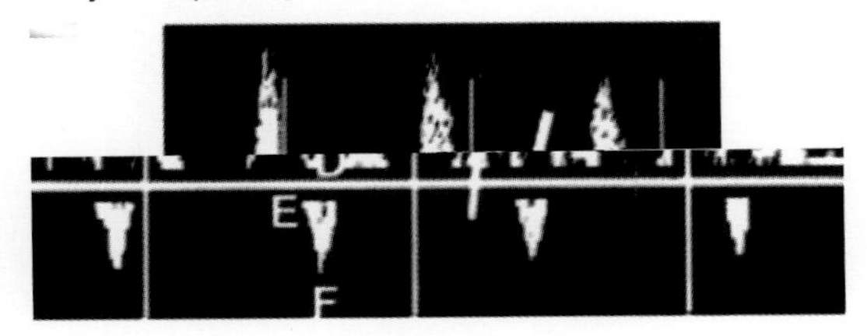

FIGURE 1.4B

After exercise, a pronounced forward-flow component appears in diastole (white arrow) due to the decrease in peripheral resistance. The spectral pattern is intermediate between A and C

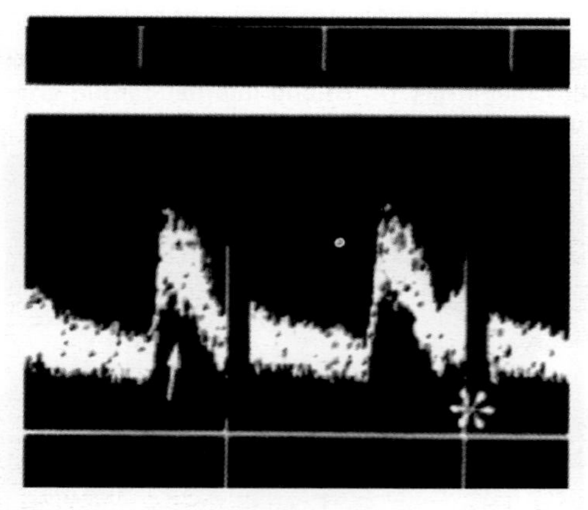

FIGURE 1.4C

Low peripheral resistance. The spectrum displays a high diastolic forward flow and less pulsatility than in A and B (parenchymal artery pattern). The empty systolic window (arrow) indicates undisturbed flow. Periodic refreshing of the color Duplex image creates a brief, intermittent void in the spectral waveform (*)

PULSATILITY

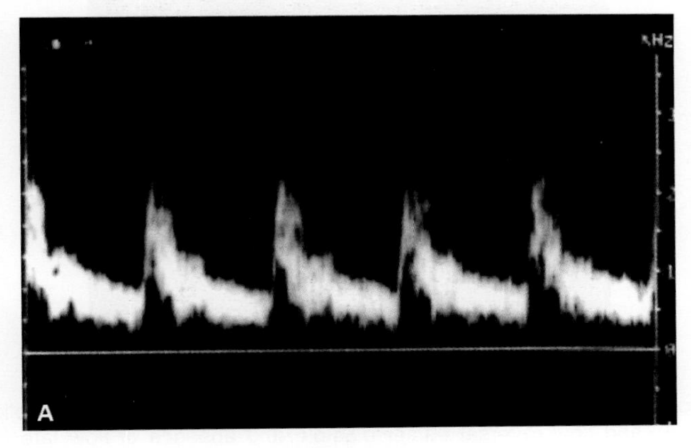

FIGURE 1.5A

Low pulsatility is indicated by a broad systolic peak and persistent forward flow throughout diastole (e.g. internal carotid artery)

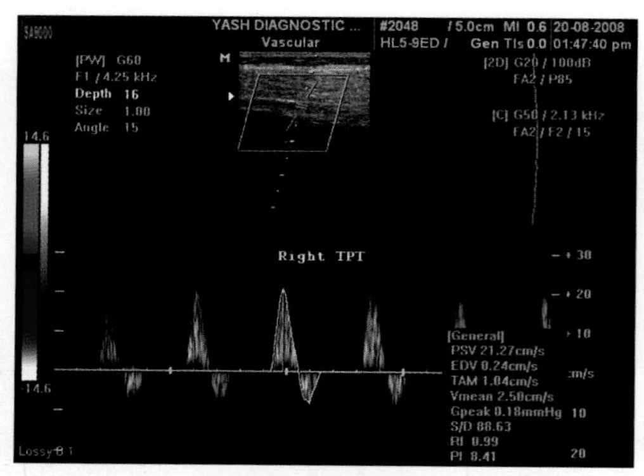

FIGURE 1.5B

Moderate pulsatility is indicated by a tall, sharp and narrow systolic peak, and flow reversal earlier diastole and absence of flow late in diastole

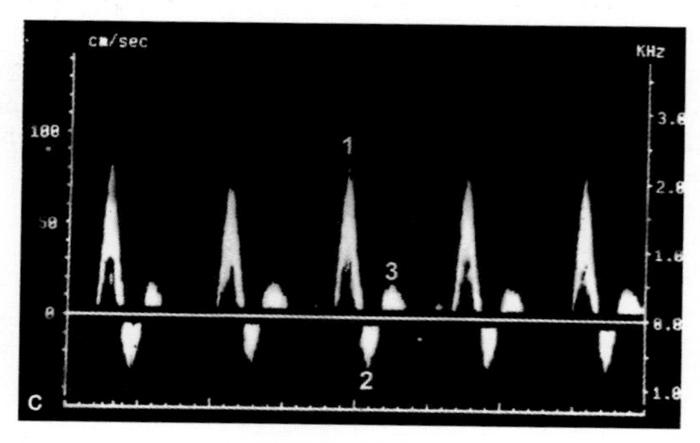

FIGURE 1.5C

High pulsatility, classic example is triphasic pattern: The first phase (1) is systole, and the second phase (2) is brief diastolic flow reversal and the third phase (3) is diastolic forward flow and relatively little diastolic flow

LAMINAR FLOW

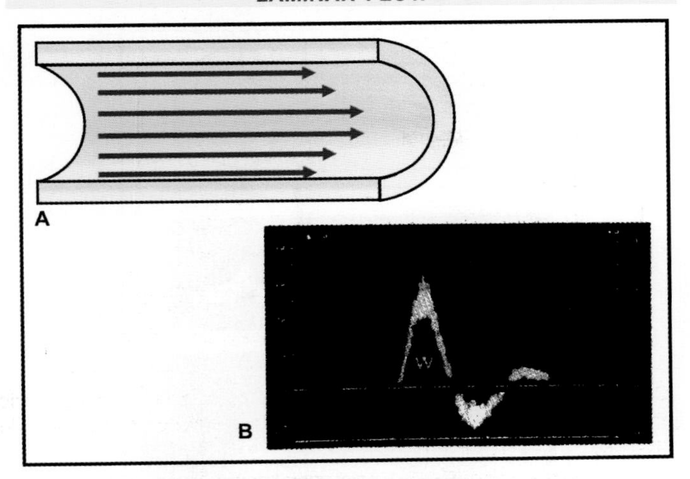

FIGURES 1.6 A and B

(A) Illustration of parallel lines of blood cell movement, (B) Doppler spectrum during laminar flow. At all times, the blood cells are moving at similar velocities. As a result, the spectrum is a thin line that encloses a well-defined black "window" (W)

DISTURBED FLOW

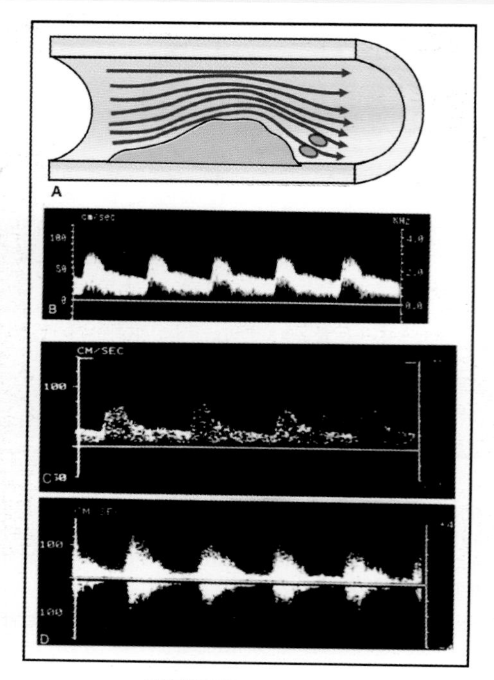

FIGURES 1.7A to D

(A) Disturbed flow illustration, (B) Minor flow disturbance is indicated by spectral broadening at peak systole and through diastole, (C) Moderate flow disturbance causes fill-in of the spectral window (D) Severe flow disturbance is characterized by spectral fill-in, poor definition of spectral borders, and simultaneous forward and reversed flow. The audible Doppler signal has a loud, gruff character when flow is severely disturbed

NORMAL BIFURCATION FLOW DISTURBANCE

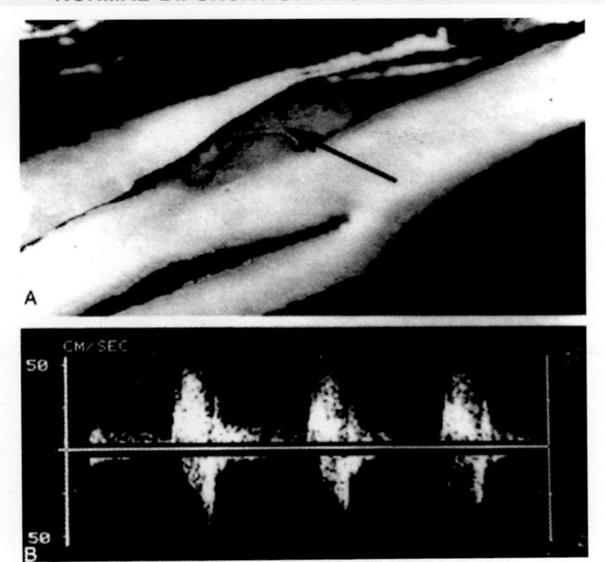

FIGURES 1.8A and B

(A) Flow reversal in the bulbous portion of the common and internal carotid arteries causes localized flow reversal (arrow), (B) Simultaneous forward and reverse flow is evident in the bulbous region on the Doppler spectrum indicating turbulence due to changes in diameter of vessel

ALIASING ARTEFACT

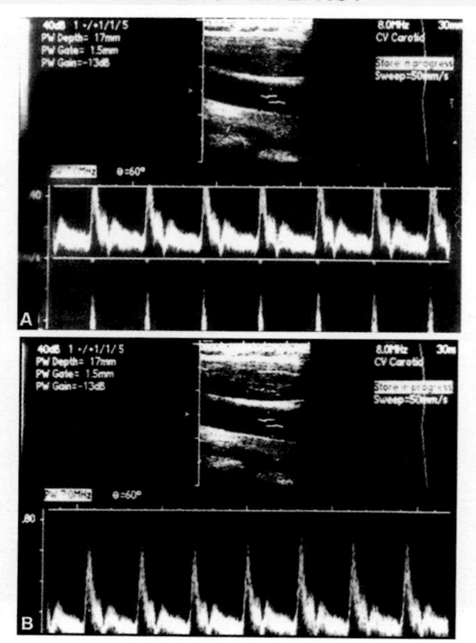

FIGURES 1.9A and B

(A) Shows aliasing artefact caused by improper settings. Aliasing is said to occur when the PSV portion of the Doppler spectrum is represented on the other side of the baseline or occur if the frequency shift measured at very high flow velocities exceeds the Nyquist limit of (Pulse Repetition Frequency) PRF/2, the corresponding portion of the spectral waveform will be cut off and displayed on the opposite side of the spectrum, (B) Correction of aliasing should be achieved by lowering baseline on the machine followed by increasing the velocity scale to get the optimal Doppler trace. Also can be corrected by increasing the PRF or by using the lower frequency transducer or increase the beam angle (α) within limits

COLOR FLOW SCHEMES

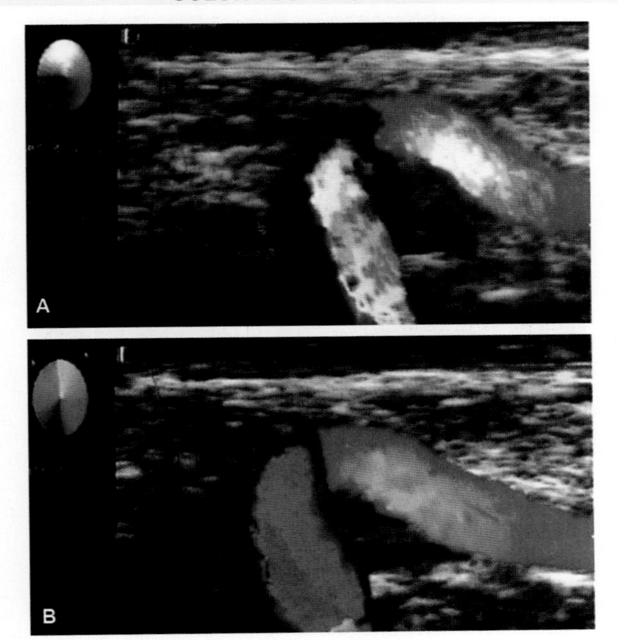

FIGURES 1.10 A and B

Color flow schemes. A variety of color schemes are used in color Doppler instruments.
(A) With this scheme, progressive increase in the frequency shift changes the image color from red to pink to white, or from dark blue to light blue to white, depending on the flow direction, (B) With this scheme, the color changes from red to yellow or from blue to green, as the frequency shift increases

COLOR AMPLITUDE IMAGE OF A KIDNEY

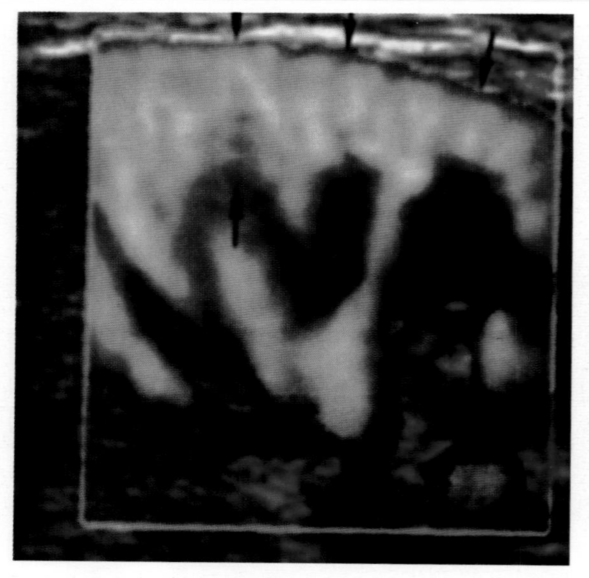

FIGURE 1.11

Conventional color flow image shows the presence of a range of frequency shifts in the cortical region of the kidney and noise in the tissue. The letter is represented by color of non-vascular origin

POWER DOPPLER IN CRANIAL VASCULATURE

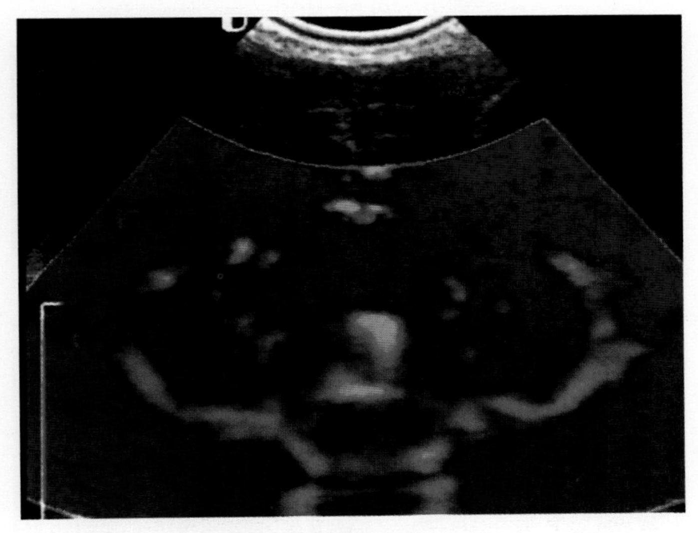

FIGURE 1.12

This power Doppler image of the cranial vasculature uses a blue background which enhances flow detection because noise is converted to a uniform blue color

QUANTITATIVE SPECTRAL WAVEFORM IN POWER DOPPLER MODE

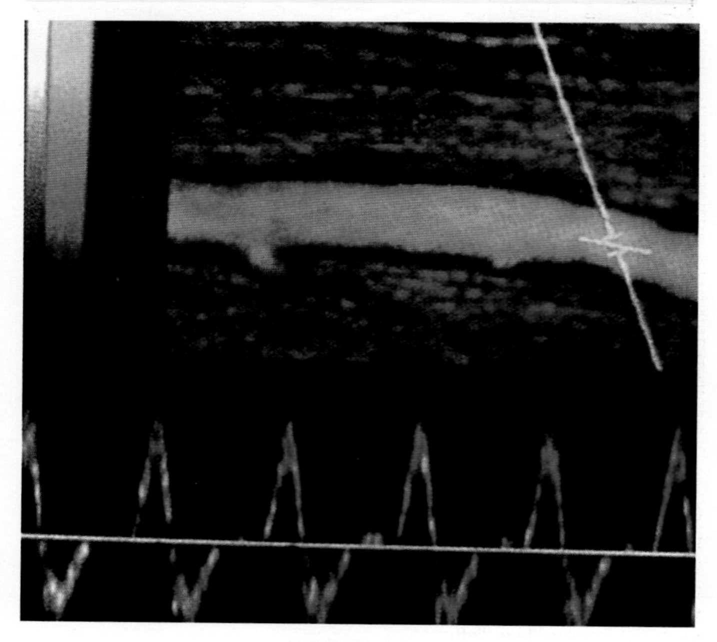

FIGURE 1.13

Quantitative spectral information can be obtained in power Doppler mode. It has the advantage of being less angle dependent and free from aliasing artefact

LOCAL EFFECTS OF ARTERIAL STENOSIS

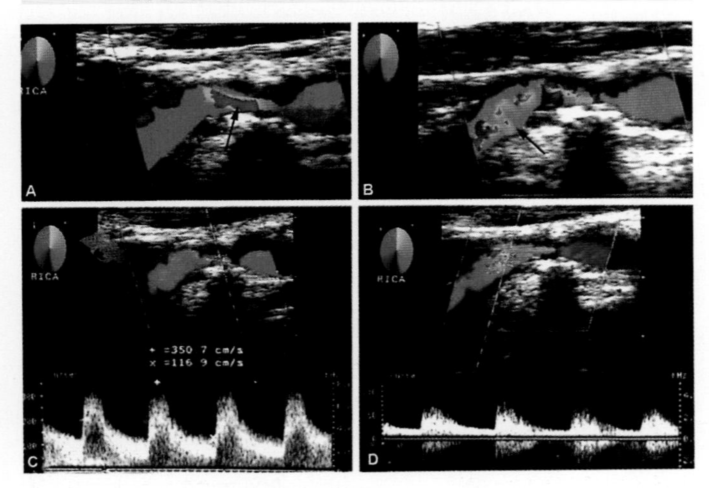

FIGURES 1.14A to D

(A) High velocities present in the narrowed portion of the arterial lumen generate an area of aliasing (arrow) within the stenotic lumen, (B) Disturbed flow in the post-stenotic area generates a mixture of colors (arrow), (C) Doppler spectral analysis shows markedly elevated velocity at peak systole (350.7 cm/sec) and end diastole (116.9 cm/sec), (D) Severe flow disturbance is evident in the post-stenotic region, as indicated by simultaneous forward and reverse flow, spectrum fill-in, and poor definition of the spectrum margins

Relationship of PSV with reduction cross-sectional area of stenosis

PSV	*Reduction in cross-sectional area*
<2.5	0-49%
>2.5	50-74%
>5.5	75-99%

Always remember – the criteria for stenosis

a) In the Doppler spectrum:
- Flattened systolic upstroke
- Intrastenotic flow acceleration
- Filling-in of the spectral window (due to turbulence)
- Reduced V peak farther downstream

b) In color flow:
- Visible plaque
- Bright stenotic jet or aliasing
- Poststenotic turbulence or flow reversal near the vessel wall

Please note the common problems

		Because of	Always do
Low signal amplitudes or poor color encoding	(a)	Beam angle>60°	Use more oblique probe angle
	(b)	B-mode gain too high	Reduce B-mode gain
	(c)	Color gain too low	Increase color signal gain
	(d)	PRF too high (in veins)	Decrease PRF
	(e)	Wall filter too high (in veins)	Reduce color wall filter
Doppler trace from peripheral arteries shows normal triphasic pattern but is above the baseline		Hyperemia after physical exertion, causing decrease in peripheral resistance	Rest the patient at least 10 min and repeat the examination
Aliasing despite normal B-mode and pulsed Doppler		Too low PRF	Increase the PRF or shift the baseline
Doppler fills in with normal audio signal and flow velocities			The background appears black (free of noise)
Spectral window in pulsed		Too high PW gain	Reduce PW gain
Low velocities despite normal color image		Faulty angle correction	Realign the angle correct bar parallel to the vessel axes

WAVEFORM IN STENOSIS

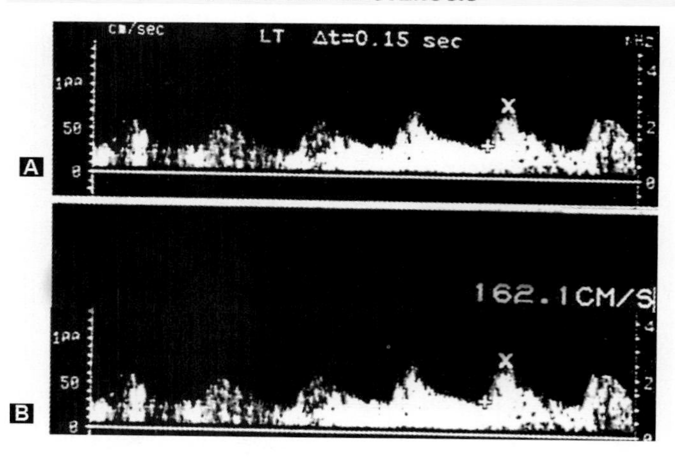

FIGURES 1.15A and B

(A) The acceleration time is prolonged (0.15 sec) in the left kidney due to severe proximal renal artery stenosis. Acceleration time is defined as the time in seconds taken by the blood flow to reach the PSV from the baseline, (B) Severely damped dorsalis pedis artery waveform distal to femoral/popliteal artery occlusion

SPECTRAL WAVEFORM IN STENOSIS

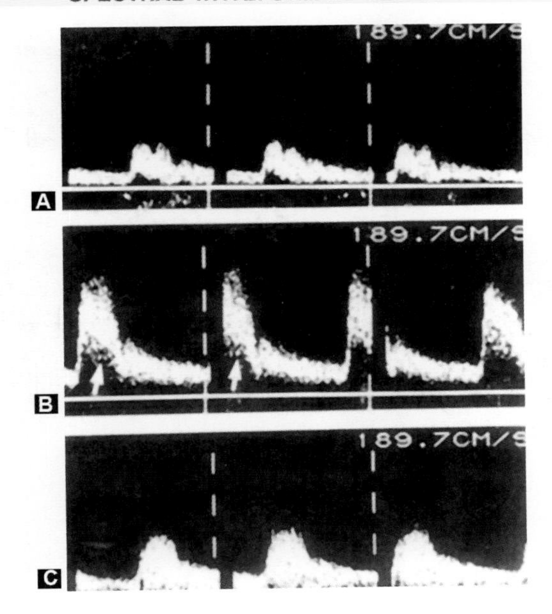

FIGURES 1.16A to C

(A) Prestenotic spectrum from common carotid artery shows low systolic and diastolic velocity with filling of the spectral window, (B) Intrastenotic spectrum shows a mark elevation of flow velocity indicating turbulence, (C) Poststenotic spectrum also shows filling of the systolic window with broader and higher systolic peak than prestenotic area

Chapter Two

Craniocervical Doppler

COLOR DOPPLER FLOW IN CCA

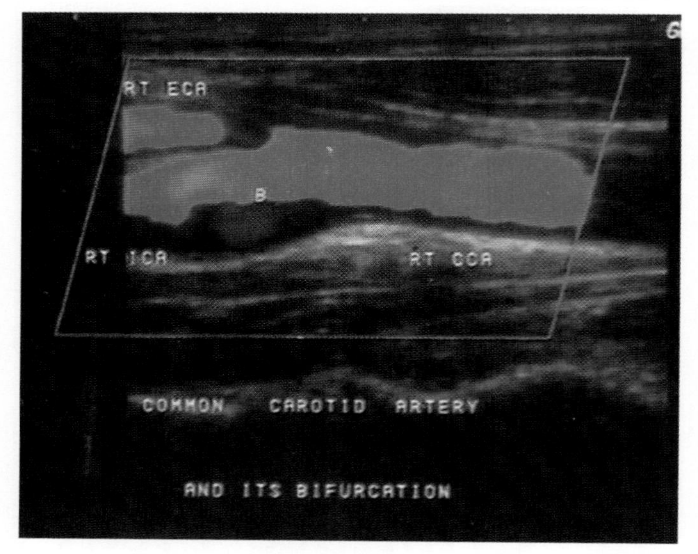

FIGURE 2.1

Normal longitudinal color Doppler flow image of the common carotid artery and its bifurcation with flow reversal tone (*blue area*) appearing at early systole or peak systole in the region of carotid bulb

DOPPLER WAVEFORM IN ECA

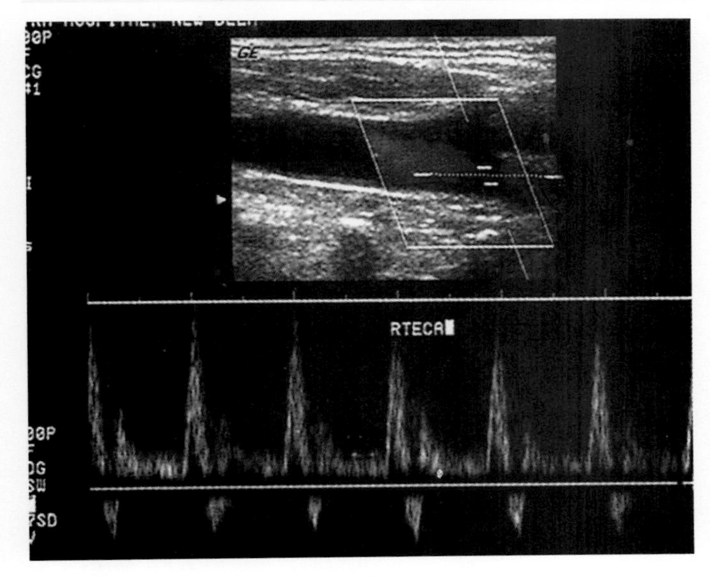

FIGURE 2.2

Doppler waveform of normal external carotid artery showing triphasic waveform characteristic of arteries supplying muscular bed; high pulsatility pattern

DOPPLER WAVEFORM IN ICA

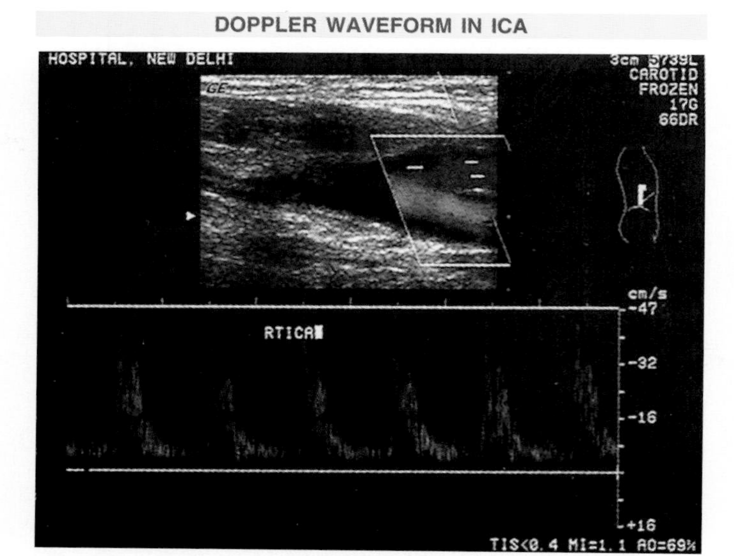

FIGURE 2.3

Normal Doppler waveform of internal carotid artery with broad peak, persistent forward flow during diastole; a low pulsatility pattern. Spectral window can also be appreciated

PULSE DOPPLER WAVEFORM IN CCA

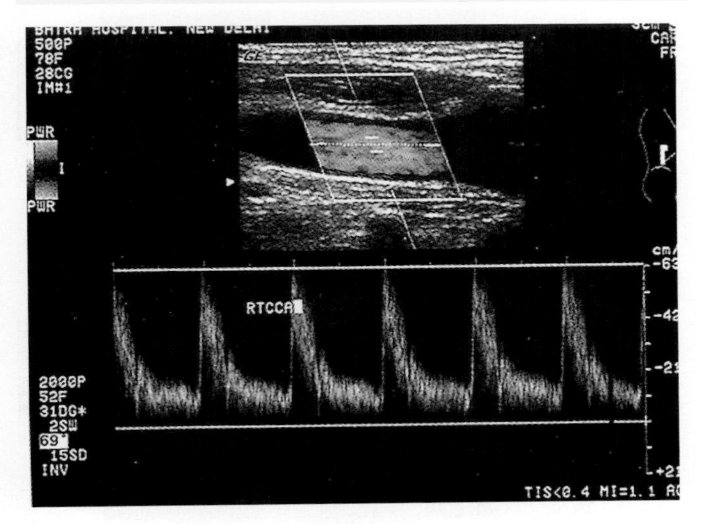

FIGURE 2.4

Pulse Doppler waveform of normal common carotid artery shows sharp systolic peak with antegrade flow during diastole; a low pulsatility pattern. The systolic peak is sharper than that of ICA and diastolic flow is less than ICA

CDFI IN CCA

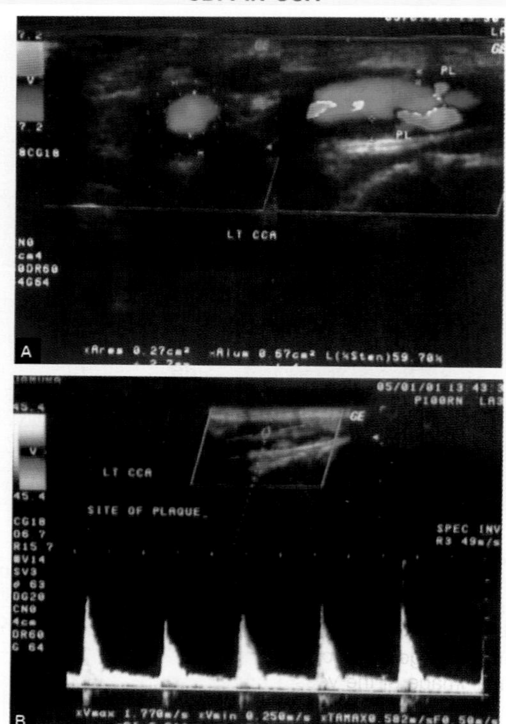

FIGURES 2.5A and B

(A) CDFI of the common carotid artery shows approximately 60% area stenosis as measured in a transverse scan, (B) Duplex scanning through the area of stenosis demonstrates increased peak systolic velocity, consistent with > 60% luminal narrowing (stenosis)

INTIMA-MEDIA THICKNESS MEASUREMENT

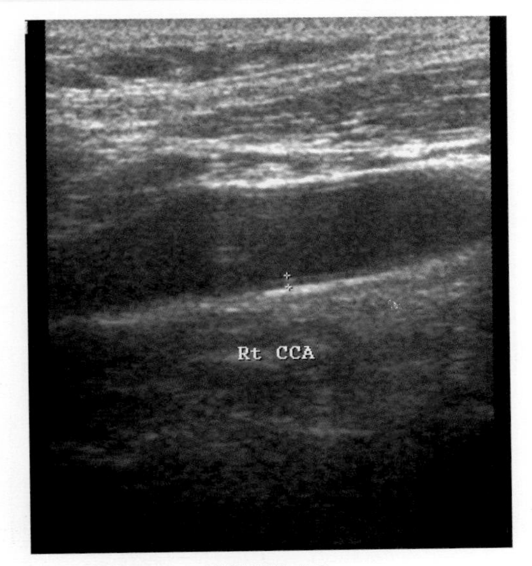

FIGURE 2.6

Gray scale image showing how to measure the intima-media thickness in carotid artery, i.e. the distance from the innermost echogenic line to the innermost edge of the outer echogenic line. It is always measured in longitudinal image of the vessel

PLAQUE IN CCA

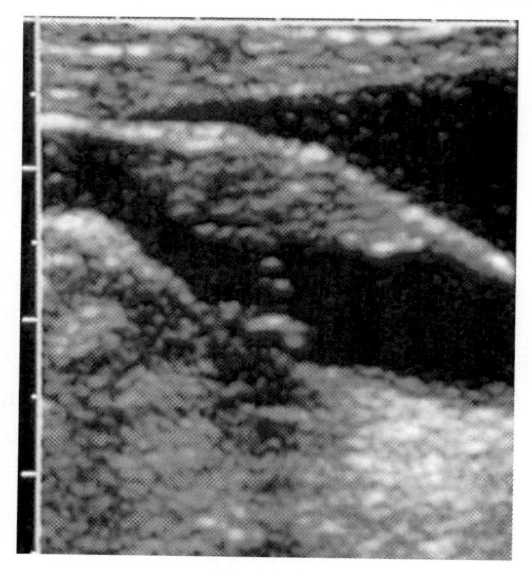

FIGURE 2.7

B-mode longitudinal image of distal common carotid artery shows a homogeneous, hypoechoic, noncalcified plaque causing significant narrowing of lumen. Such plaques are susceptible to ulceration and distal embolization

CALCIFIED PLAQUE IN CCA

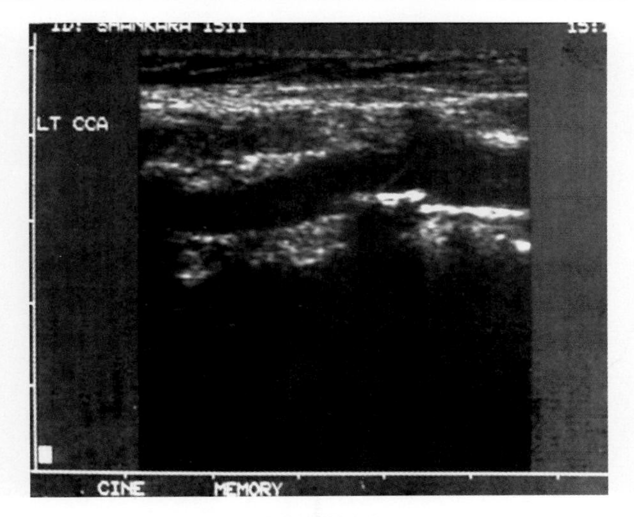

FIGURE 2.8

B-mode image of common carotid artery shows a densely calcified plaque in the posterior wall with posterior acoustic shadowing without significant narrowing of lumen. Such plaques rarely embolize

PLAQUE IN POWER DOPPLER

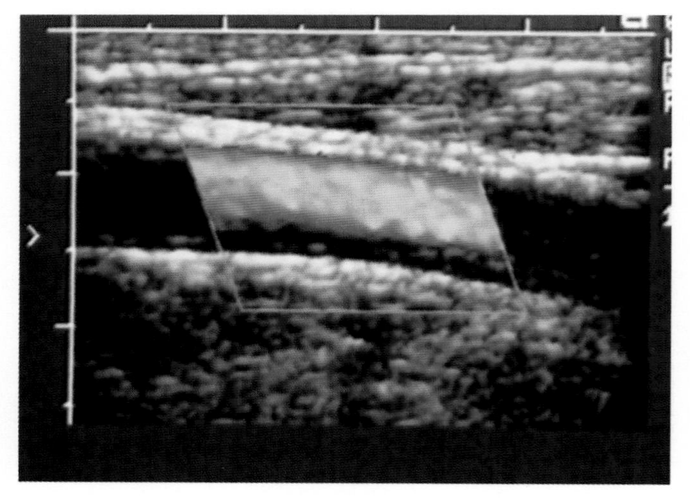

FIGURE 2.9

Power Doppler image of common carotid artery showing smooth, thin, homogeneous plaque in the posterior wall without significant luminal compromise

HYPOECHOIC PLAQUE IN CCA

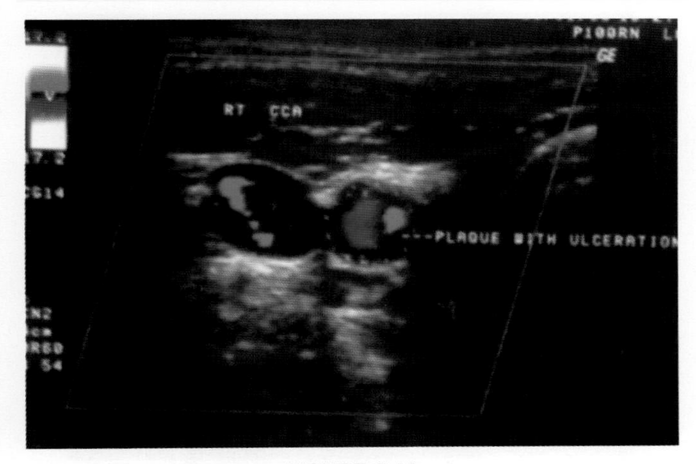

FIGURE 2.10

Transverse color Doppler image of common carotid artery shows incomplete filling of color in the vessel lumen caused by a hypoechoic plaque

SUBACUTE THROMBOSIS

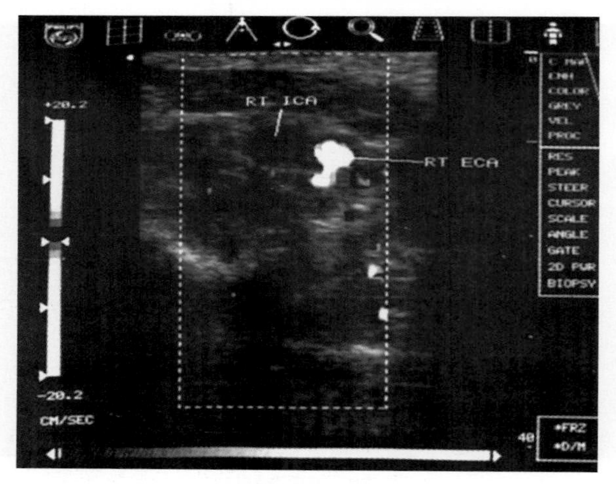

FIGURE 2.11

Transverse color flow image just above the carotid bifurcation shows complete lack of color filling of internal carotid artery with a hypoechoic material filling the lumen suggesting subacute thrombosis

VESSEL WALL THICKENING

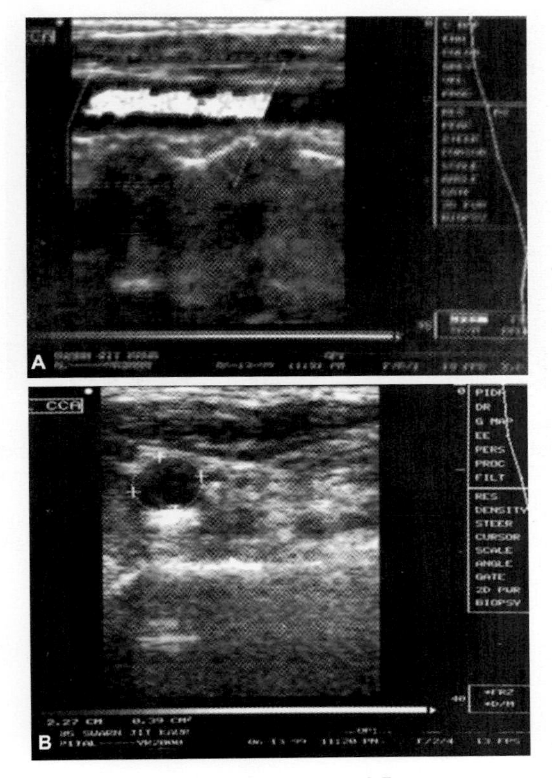

FIGURES 2.12A and B

(A) Color Doppler image of common carotid artery shows narrowing of lumen due to circumferential wall thickening, (B) Transverse section showing circumferential wall thickening

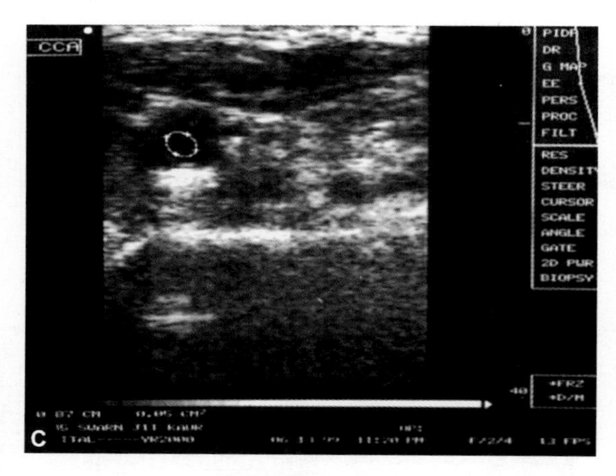

FIGURE 2.12C

Measurement of area of vessel and residual lumen by electronic calipers shows 87% area stenosis. This figure also demonstrates the method of measuring the degree of stenosis

CIRCLE OF WILLIS

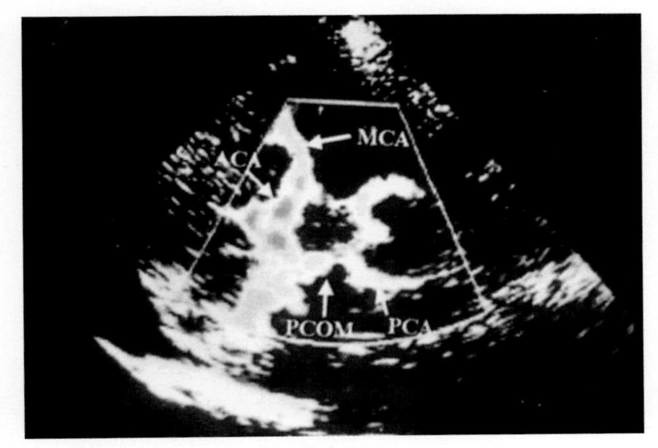

FIGURE 2.13

Color Duplex TCD image (transtemporal window) in gray tone shows circle of Willis including middle cerebral artery (MCA), anterior cerebral artery (ACA), posterior cerebral artery (PCA) and posterior communicating artery (PCOM)

MIDDLE CEREBRAL ARTERY

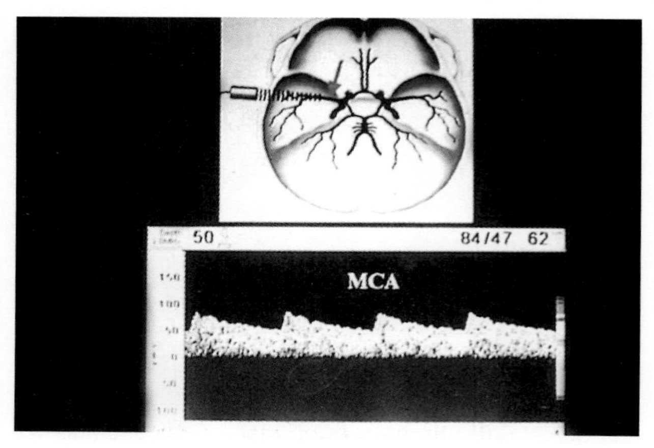

FIGURE 2.14

Picture depicting middle cerebral artery insonation through transtemporal approach and spectral waveform from the artery showing low resistance waveform with flow towards the transducer

INTERNAL CAROTID ARTERY (TERMINAL PORTION)

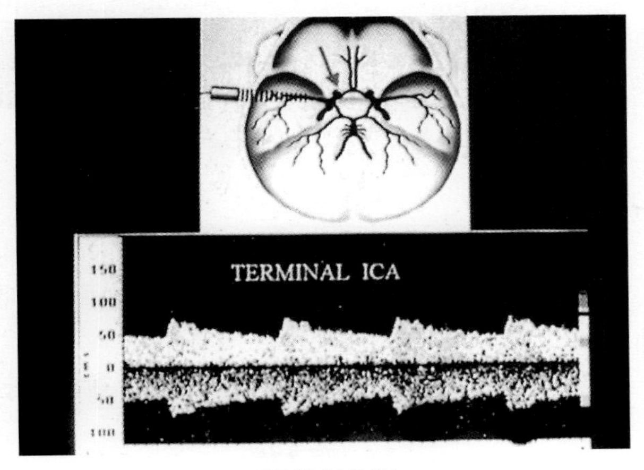

FIGURE 2.15

Picture depicting terminal internal carotid artery insonation through transtemporal approach and spectral waveform from the artery showing typical bi-directional flow

ANTERIOR CEREBRAL ARTERY

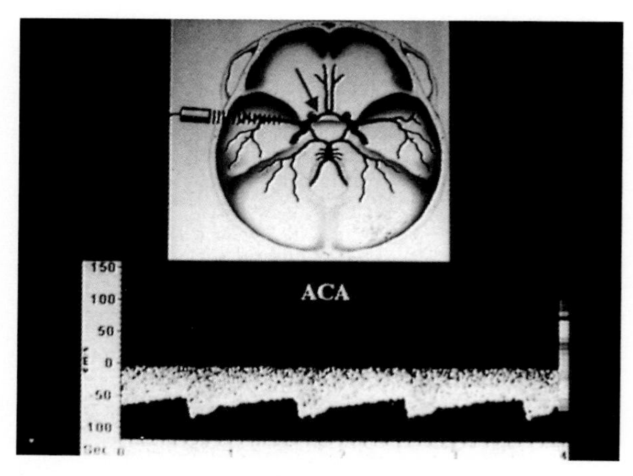

FIGURE 2.16

Picture depicting anterior cerebral artery insonation through trans-temporal approach and spectral waveform from the artery showing low resistance waveform with flow away from the transducer

SUBARACHNOID HEMORRHAGE - VASOSPASM

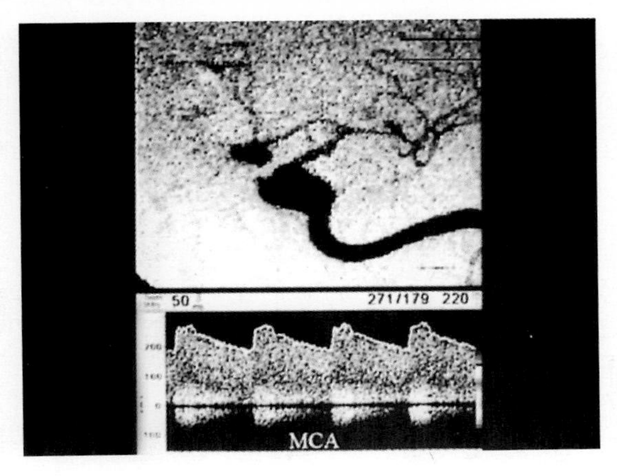

FIGURE 2.17

IADSA image in a case with subarachnoid hemorrhage showing aneurysm arising from anterior communicating artery with marked spasm of internal carotid, middle cerebral and anterior cerebral arteries. Spectral waveform from middle cerebral artery shows increased velocities (220 cm/s) and spectral broadening, diagnostic of spasm

SUBARACHNOID HEMORRHAGE WITH VASOSPASM – SERIAL STUDIES

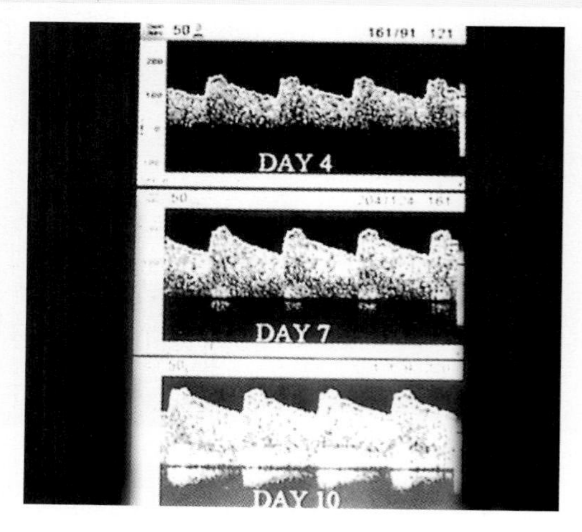

FIGURE 2.18

Spectral waveforms from left middle cerebral artery in a case with subarachnoid hemorrhage shows mildly increased velocity (121 cm/s) at day 4. Progressive increase in velocity (161 cm/s) seen at day 7 and day 10 (220 cm/s). This patient developed ipsilateral middle cerebral artery infarct. Therefore, evolution of vasospasm can be observed by TCD and rapid rise in flow velocities can be a warning signal for significant vasospasm and subsequent infarction

MIDDLE CEREBRAL ARTERY STENOSIS

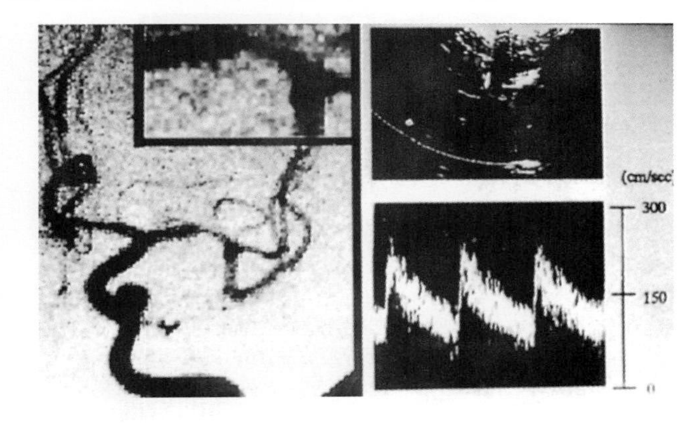

FIGURE 2.19

IADSA image in a patient with transient ischemic attacks in left middle cerebral artery shows significant stenosis of middle cerebral artery. Special waveform (shown on the left side) had shown significantly increased velocities (200 cm/s) in this artery

MOYA-MOYA DISEASE

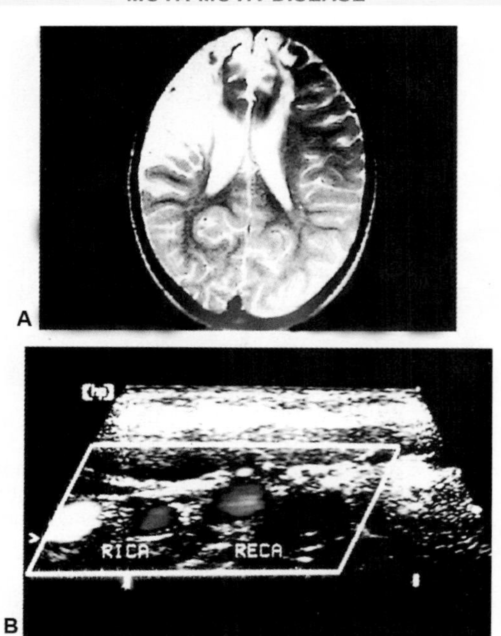

FIGURES 2.20A and B

Axial T2-weighted image (A) in a child with repeated strokes shows multiple infarcts. Color Doppler image (B) in neck region shows internal carotid artery is smaller than external carotid artery

MOYA-MOYA DISEASE

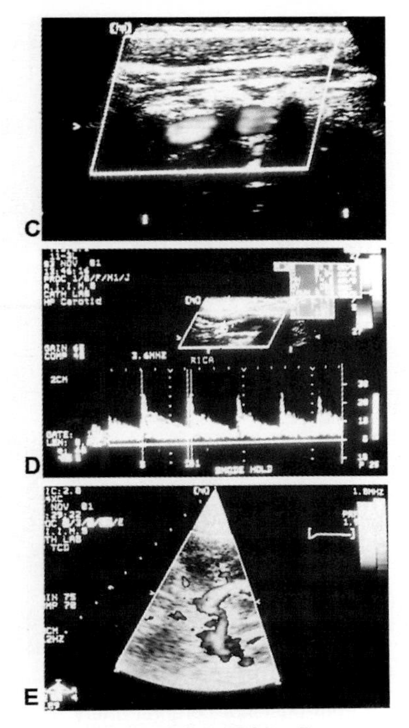

FIGURES 2.20C to E

Vertebral artery is dilated (C), Spectral waveform from cervical internal carotid artery (D) shows decreased flow velocities (23 cm/s) due to decreased flow, Color TCD image (E) shows dilated posterior cerebral arteries in contrast to poorly visualized middle and anterior cerebral arteries

MOYA-MOYA DISEASE

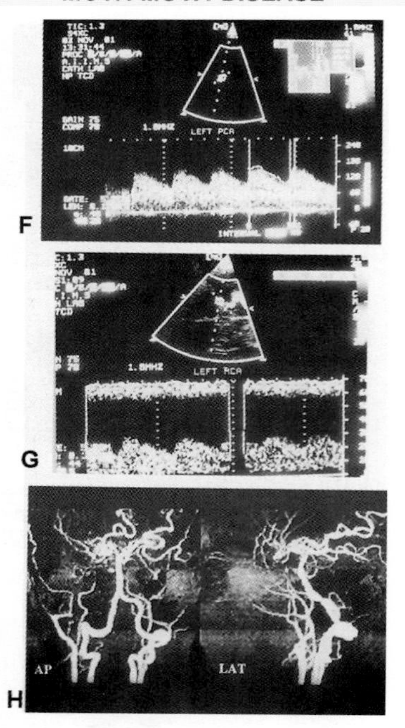

FIGURES 2.20F to H

Spectral waveform from posterior cerebral artery (F) shows increased flow velocities (160 cm/s) because it is providing collateral flow while middle cerebral artery (G) shows decreased flow velocity (28 cm/s) because of the proximal obstruction. These findings considered together are consistent with B/L intracranial internal carotid artery stenosis / occlusion (Moya-Moya pattern). MRA (H) confirms the diagnosis. This case illustrates the need to evaluate the extracranial arteries for proper interpretation of TCD findings

CERVICAL INTERNAL CAROTID ARTERY BLOCK

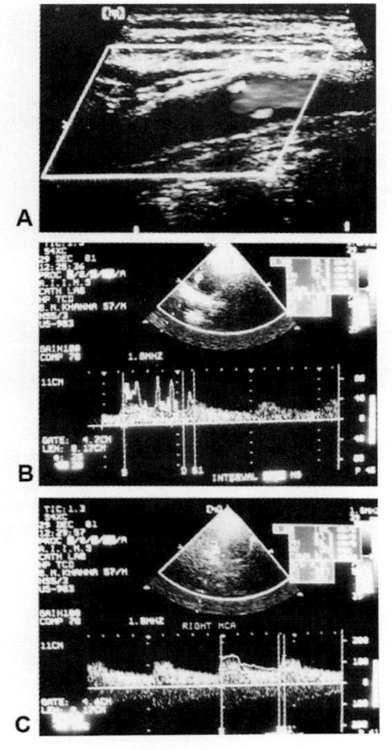

FIGURES 2.21A to C

Intracranial hemodynamic effect: Color Doppler images (A) of left cervical internal carotid artery showing block in its proximal portion. TCD examination shows decreased velocity (39 cm/s) and therefore reduced flow in left middle cerebral artery (B) as compared to the contralateral (C) middle cerebral artery (102 cm/s)

MICROEMBOLI

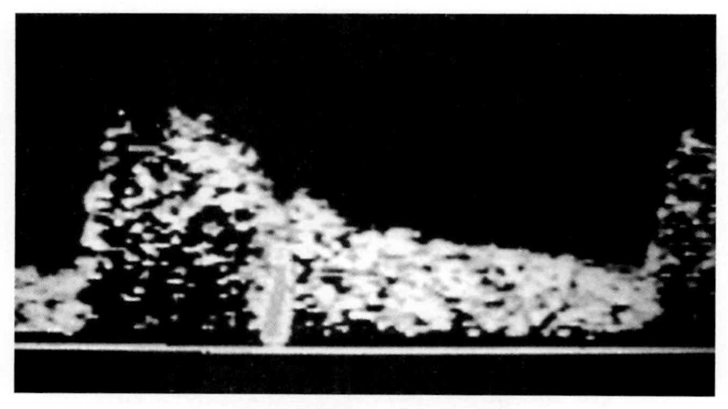

FIGURE 2.22

Detection of middle cerebral artery embolus (bright signal) in a patient with internal carotid artery plaque

TRAUMA-RAISED INTRACRANIAL PRESSURE

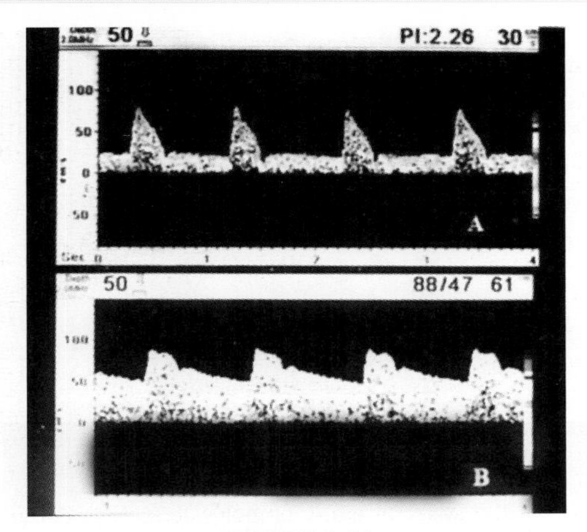

FIGURE 2.23

Spectral waveform image of middle cerebral artery (A) in a case with significant head trauma shows decreased diastolic flow while the systolic velocities are well maintained (increased pulsatility). This finding indicates raised intracranial pressure in this clinical setting. Normal spectral waveform (B) is shown below for comparison

BIRTH ASPHYXIA

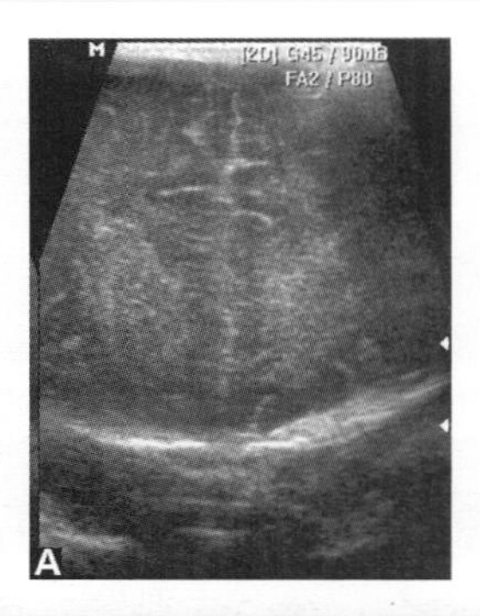

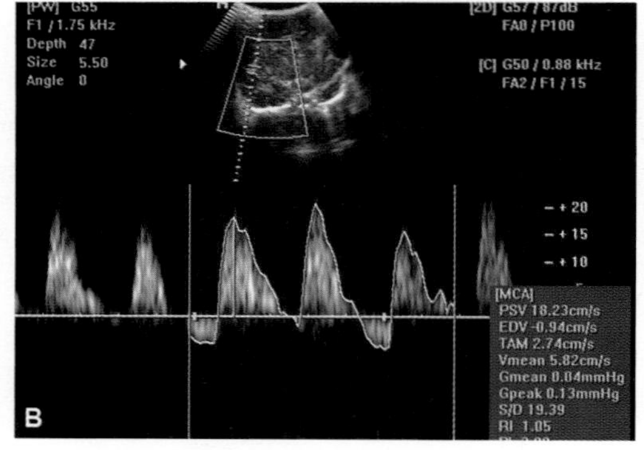

FIGURES 2.24A and B

(A) Gray scale image shows bilateral echogenic caudate nucleus in a neonate with history of birth asphyxia, (B) Duplex Doppler through middle cerebral artery shows reverse diastolic component suggestive of severe cerebral vascular compromise. Cerebral vessels should always have antegrade diastolic flow with low pulsatility pattern

THINGS TO REMEMBER

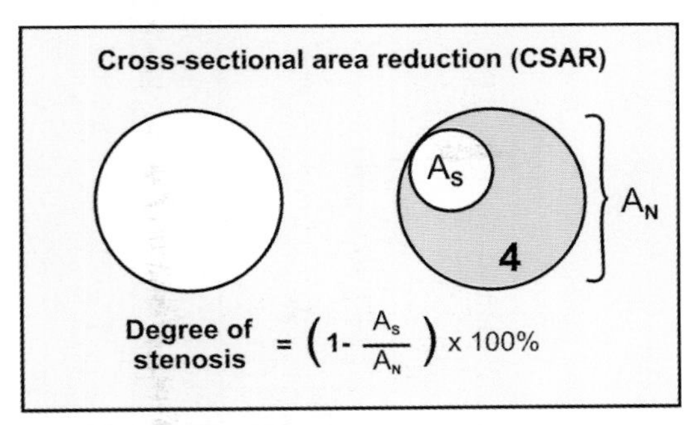

Quantifying internal carotid artery stenosis: The local degree of stenosis can be calculated in transverse image by measuring the cross-sectional area of intrastenosis, color filler residual lumen (A_S) and relating it to original vascular cross section at the site of disease (A_N).

Criteria to measure % of Internal carotid stenosis					
Criteria: % stenosis	*Intrastenotic PSV*	*Intrastenotic F*	*Intrastenotic spectrum*	*Poststenotic spectrum*	*Flow reversal in ophthalmic artery*
<40% (not (stenotic by definition)	<120 cm/s	<4 kHz	Normal	Normal	No
40-50% (mild)	~120 cm/s	~4 kHz	Slight broadening	Normal	No
51-70% (moderate)	~200 cm/s	4-7 kHz	Broadening	PSV V diast	No
71-90% (high-grade)	~300 cm/s	>7 kHz	Reverse flow components	PSV V diast	Flow , zero flow or flow reversal
91-99% (preocclusive)	Variable	Variable	Amplitude	Variable	Frequent

Intima-Media Thickness – values for CCA measurements						
Age (years)		*Left CCA*			*Right CCA*	
	50th perc.	*75th perc.*	*95th perc.*	*50th perc.*	*75th perc.*	*95th perc.*
Male						
<35	0.61	0.67	0.78	0.59	0.66	0.75
35-44	0.67	0.74	0.86	0.64	0.71	0.85
45-54	0.72	0.81	1.03	0.68	0.75	0.96
55-64	0.77	0.89	1.15	0.74	0.84	1.05
65-74	0.86	0.96	1.39	0.85	0.95	1.20
>75	0.91	1.05	2.17	0.88	1.01	1.85
Female						
<35	0.59	0.65	0.72	0.58	0.63	0.73
35-44	0.64	0.69	0.80	0.63	0.68	0.78
45-54	0.69	0.75	0.90	0.66	0.73	0.86
55-64	0.74	0.83	1.02	0.71	0.80	0.97
65-74	0.81	0.91	1.14	0.80	0.87	1.04
>75	0.85	0.99	1.28	0.82	0.91	1.16

Normal values for circle of Willis arteries			
Arteries	*PSV (cm/s)*	*Scan angle (%)*	*Error (%)*
MCA	107 ± 14	33 ± 15	15
ACA	98 ± 15	35 ± 17	18
PCA	75 ± 17	45 ± 18	30
BA	58 ± 14	15 ± 14	3

Chapter Three

Doppler in Liver

NORMAL PORTAL VENOUS WAVEFORM

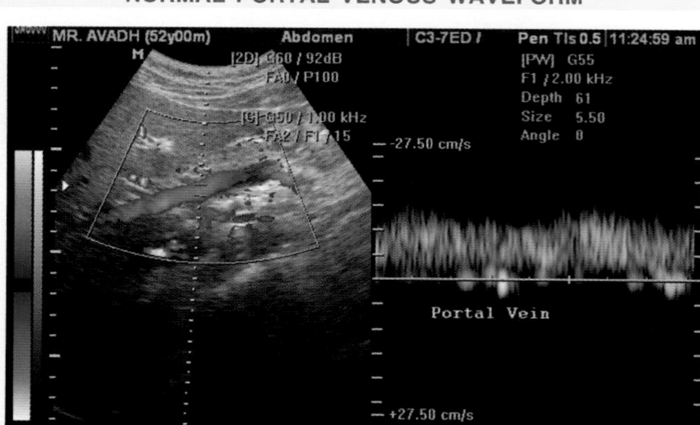

FIGURE 3.1

Duplex Doppler showing normal portal venous waveform with continuous low monophasic flow with respiratory variations

PULSED DOPPLER IN RIGHT HEPATIC VEIN

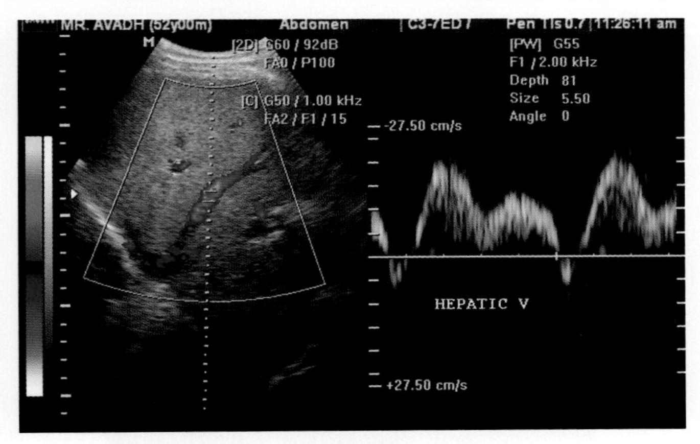

FIGURE 3.2

Pulsed Doppler tracing of right hepatic vein in a normal subject showing the characteristic three-phase profile according to the phases of the cardiac cycle and pressure changes in right atrium and inferior vena cava

CDI IN PORTAL VEIN

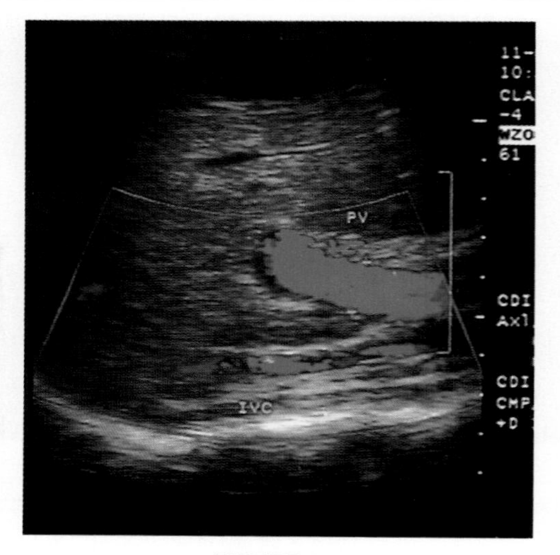

FIGURE 3.3

Color Doppler image of the porta hepatis shows dilated portal vein in a case of portal hypertension with hepatopetal flow. At porta, portal vein diameter of more than 13 mm is considered significant and more than 15 mm is considered unequivocally dilated

SPLENOPORTAL AXIS

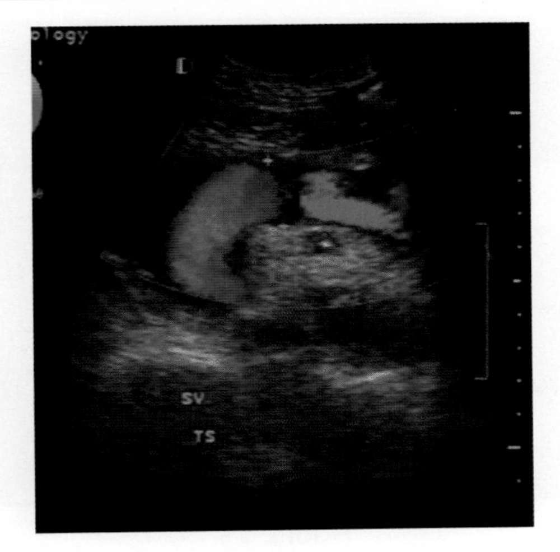

FIGURE 3.4

Color Doppler image shows grossly dilated splenoportal axis with normal direction of flow, i.e. hepatopetal flow. Splenic vein dilatation may be seen in cases of splenomegaly and is nonspecific indicator for portal hypertension

PORTAL HYPERTENSION

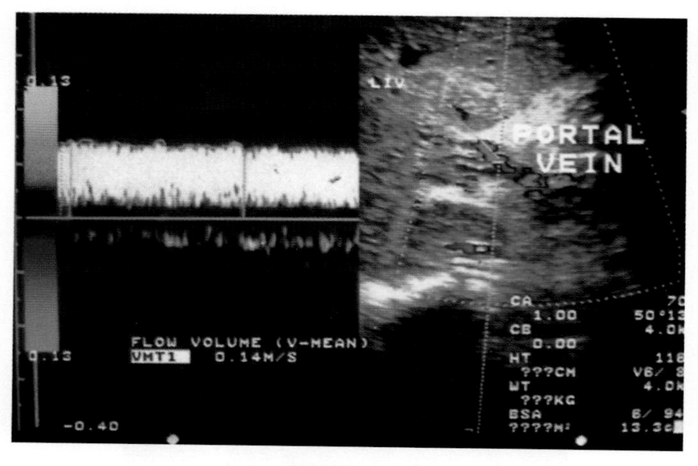

FIGURE 3.5

Duplex Doppler evaluation of portal vein showing hepatopetal portal venous flow with loss of respiratory phasicity indicative of early portal hypertension

THROMBOSED SPLENOPORTAL AXIS

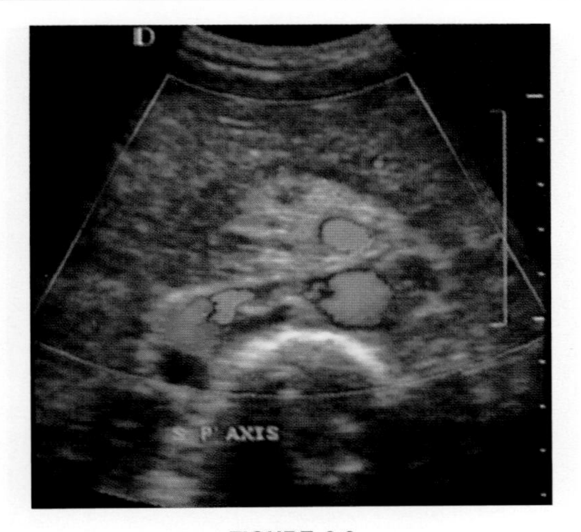

FIGURE 3.6

Color Doppler image shows heteroechoic mass filling the splenoportal axis with no detectable color flow suggestive of chronically thrombosed splenoportal axis

PORTAL CAVERNOMA

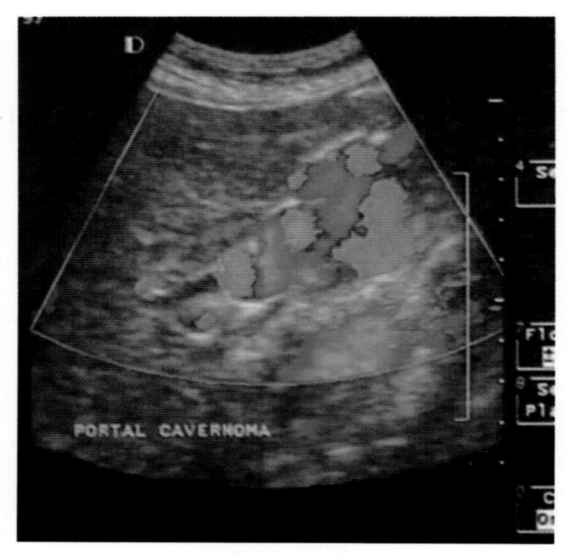

FIGURE 3.7

Color Doppler image shows portal cavernoma formation which is a characteristic sequelae of chronic main portal vein thrombosis with failure of recanalization. Hence multiple tortuous vascular channels replace the main portal vein

THROMBUS IN PORTAL VEIN

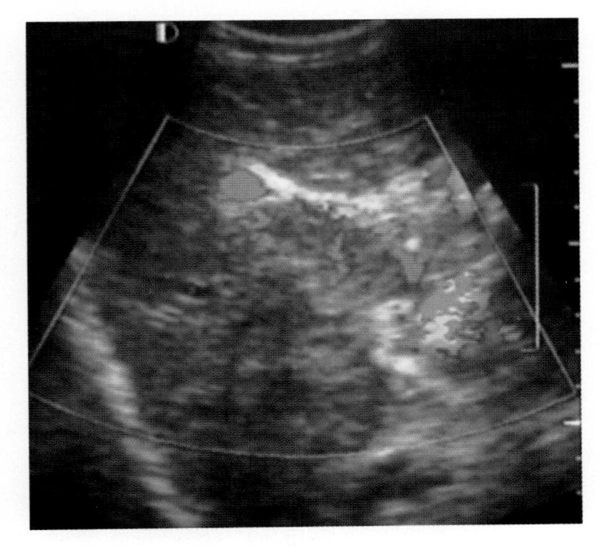

FIGURE 3.8

Color Doppler flow image shows an echogenic tumor thrombus partially occluding the portal vein. The thrombus is contiguous with a heterogeneous mass lesion in the adjacent hepatic parenchyma. Color flow is also seen within the tumor thrombus which differentiates it from bland or non-tumoral thrombus

PORTAL HYPERTENSION

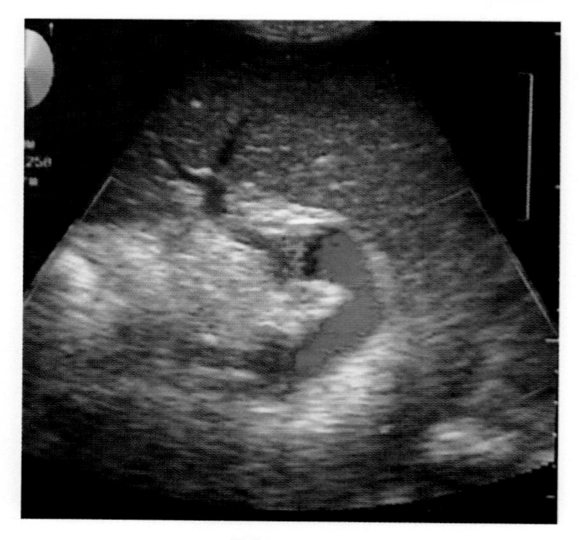

FIGURE 3.9

Color Doppler image at the splenic hilum shows dilated and tortuous splenic vein that can occur with splenomegaly secondary to any cause including portal hypertension

CDI IN CIRRHOSIS

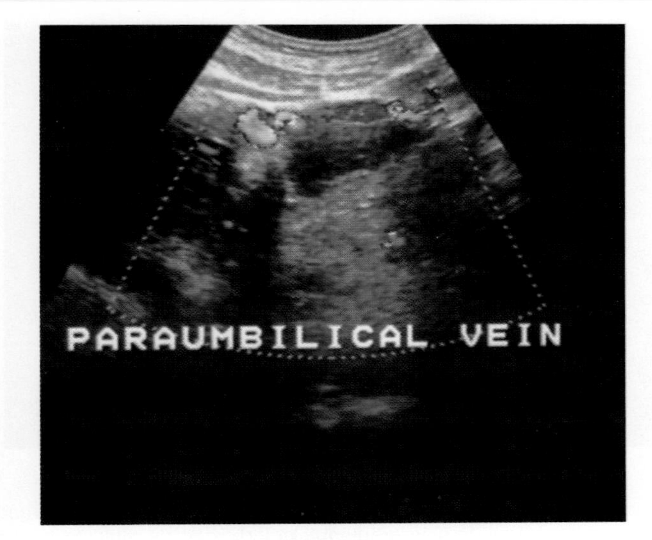

FIGURE 3.10

Color Doppler image shows patent paraumbilical vein with hepatofugal flow in a case of advanced cirrhosis suggestive of portosystemic shunting of blood

CDI IN ADVANCED CIRRHOSIS

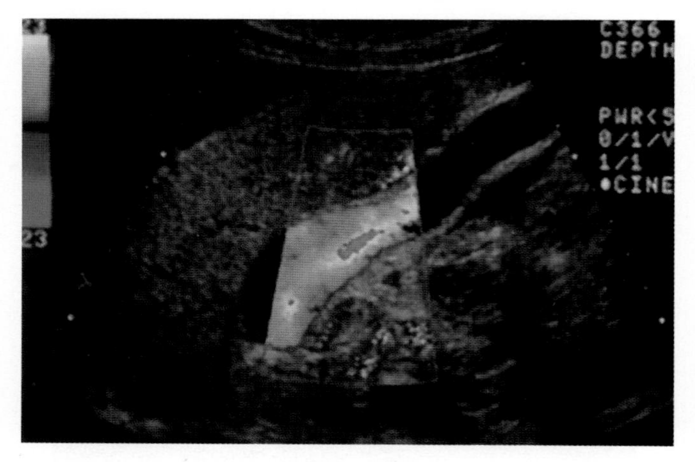

FIGURE 3.11

Color Doppler image in a patient with advanced cirrhosis shows enlarged paraumbilical venous flow gradients as indicated by multiple colors within the lumen of vein

CDI IN CIRRHOSIS

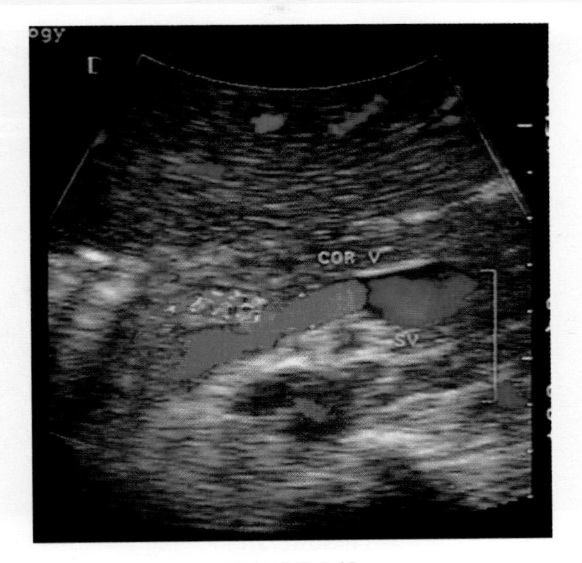

FIGURE 3.12

Color Doppler image in a known patient of cirrhosis with history of repeated variceal bleeding shows dilated coronary vein secondary to portal hypertension with hepatofugal flow

CDI IN CIRRHOSIS

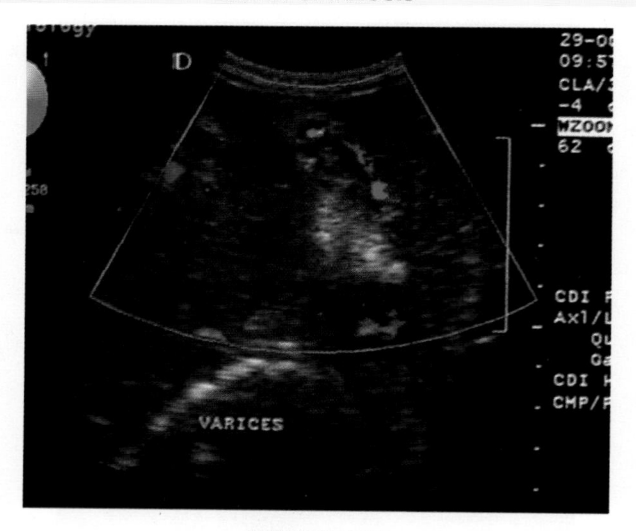

FIGURE 3.13

Color Doppler image in a known patient of cirrhosis shows tortuous varices at gastro-esophageal junction indicative of portosystemic shunting of blood

CDI IN CIRRHOSIS

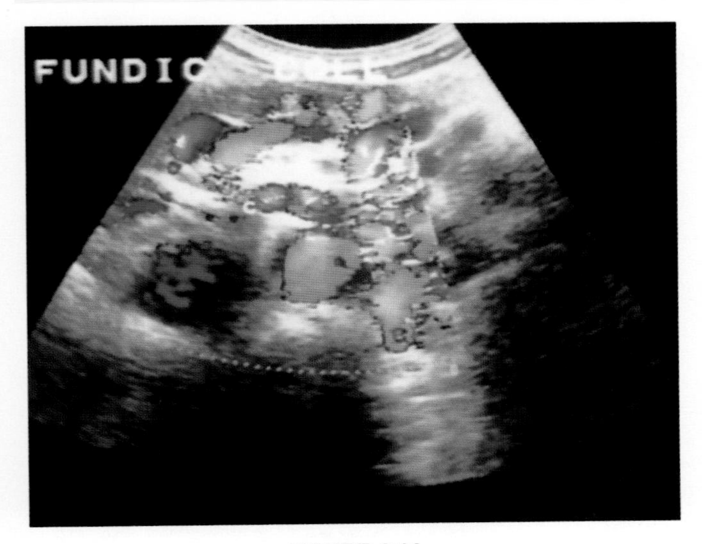

FIGURE 3.14

Color Doppler image in a known patient of cirrhosis shows voluminous collaterals at gastro-esophageal junction and at fundus of stomach (sites of portosystemic shunting of blood)

CDI IN CIRRHOSIS

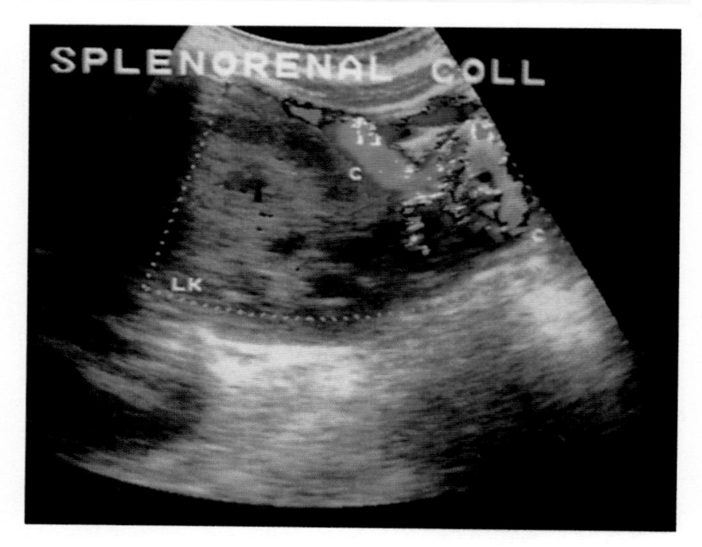

FIGURE 3.15

Color Doppler image in a known patient of cirrhosis shows splenorenal (lienorenal) collaterals indicative of portosystemic shunting of blood

CDI IN CIRRHOSIS

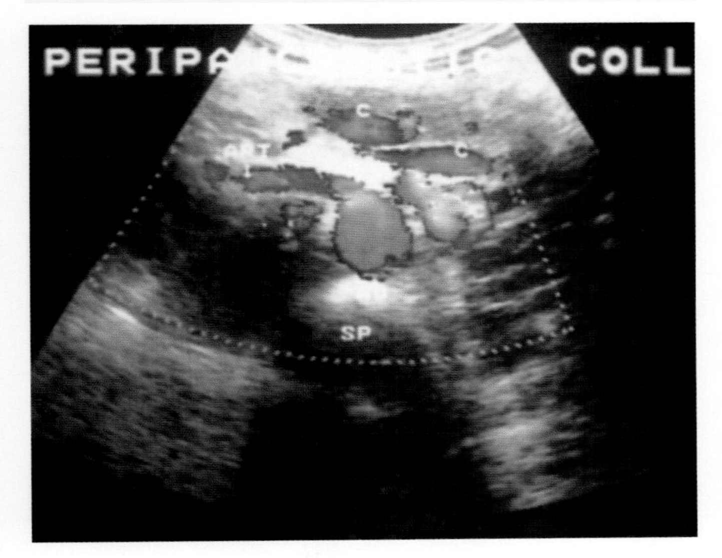

FIGURE 3.16

Color Doppler image in a known patient of cirrhosis show peripancreatic collaterals; another site of portosystemic shunting of blood

CDI IN CIRRHOSIS

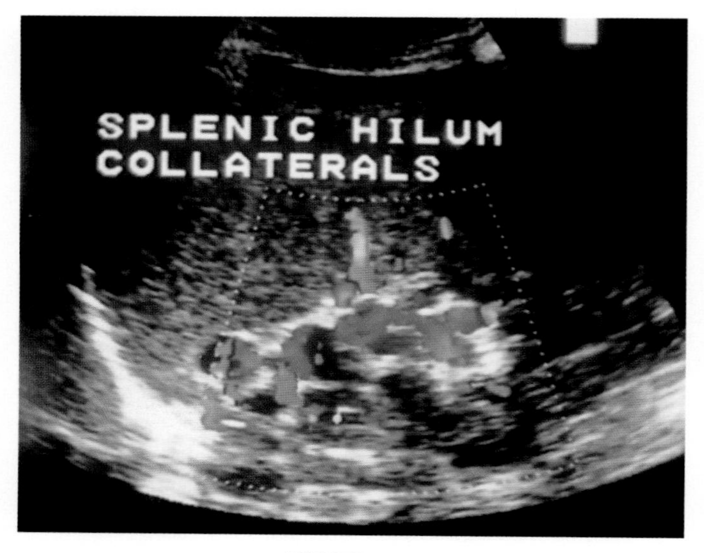

FIGURE 3.17

Color Doppler image in a known patient of cirrhosis shows splenic hilum collaterals

CDI IN LIENORENAL SHUNT

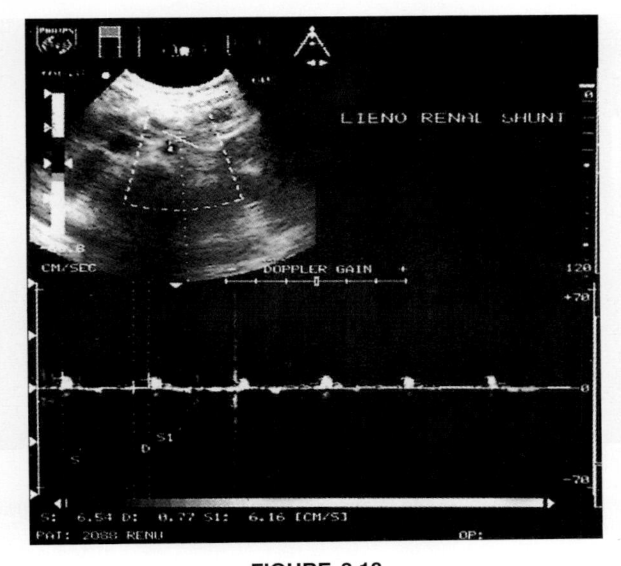

FIGURE 3.18

Duplex Doppler of lienorenal shunt showing low velocity flow

POWER DOPPLER IMAGE

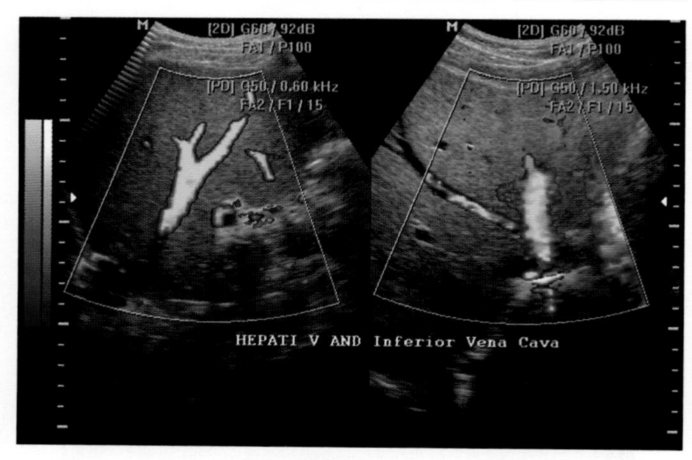

FIGURE 3.19

Hepatic veins draining into inferior vena cava (IVC) with complete filling of the lumen

DDI IN HEPATIC ABSCESS (PRE TREATMENT)

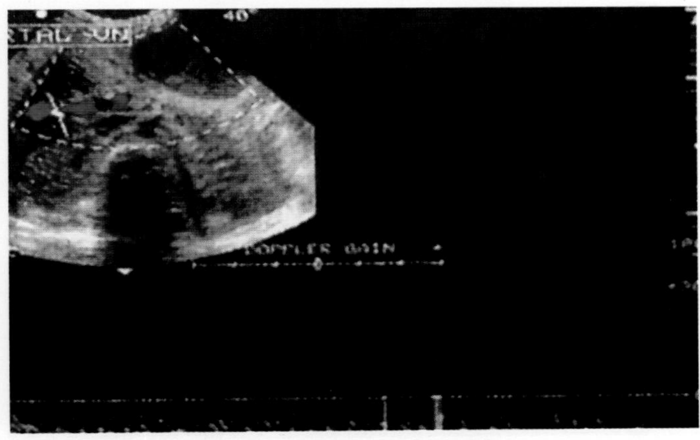

FIGURE 3.20A

Duplex Doppler image in a case of hepatic abscess before treatment showing reversal of portal flow in the anterior branch of the right portal vein

DDI IN HEPATIC ABSCESS (POST TREATMENT)

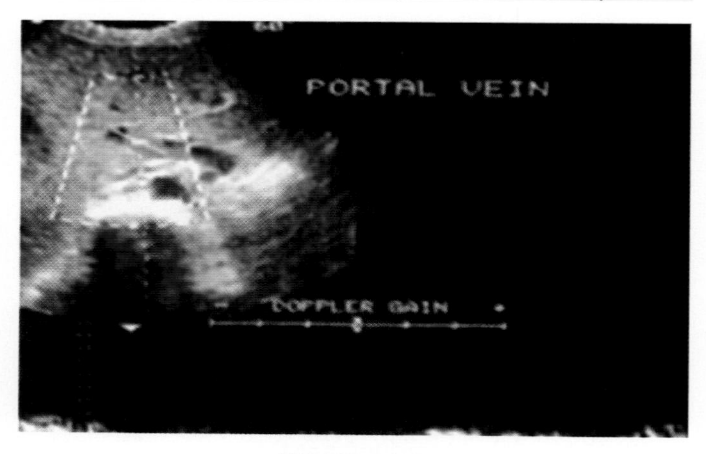

FIGURE 3.20B

Duplex Doppler US of the same case after treatment showing normalization of portal flow. Also note the change in color code of the vessel

CDF IN CARCINOMA GALLBLADDER

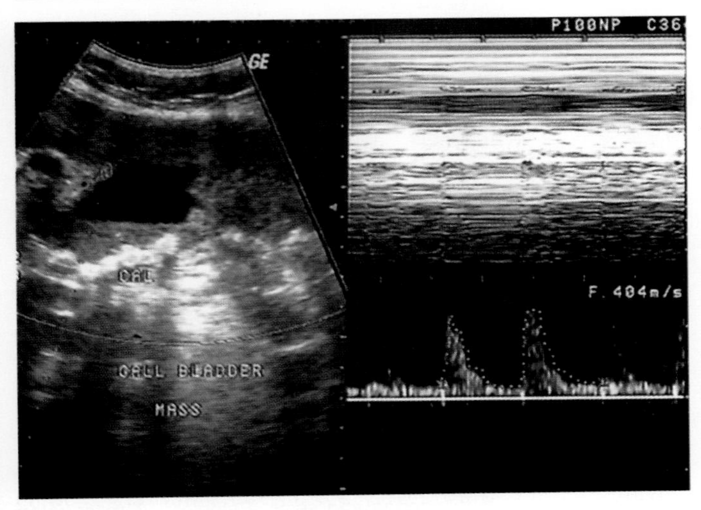

FIGURE 3.21

Color Doppler flow mapping in a case of cholelithiasis associated with carcinoma of gallbladder: Poorly defined anatomical boundary of GB. Multiple calculi in the lumen associated with mass lesion in fundus and body of GB. Anterior wall is irregularly thickened due to neoplasia and vascular study shows high pulsatility pattern suggestive of neovascularization

HEPATIC TRANSPLANT REJECTION

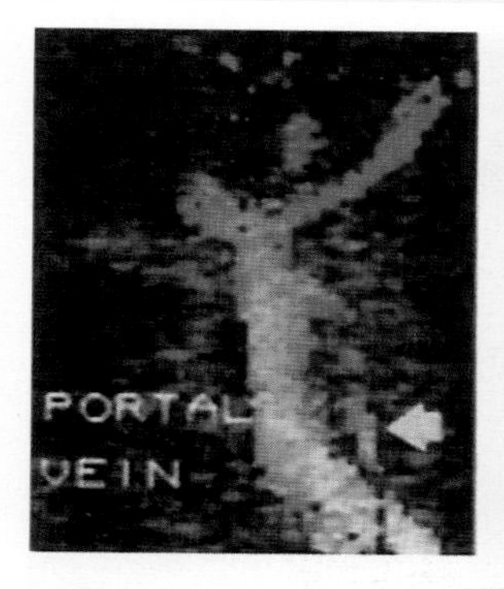

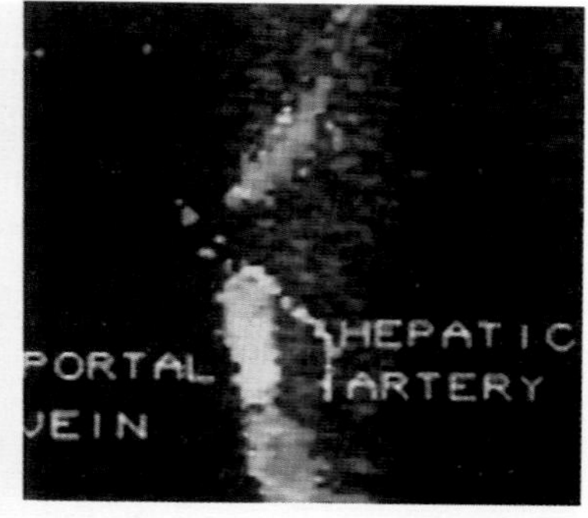

FIGURE 3.22

Severe acute hepatic transplant rejection (left) five days after transplant. There is a hepatopetal flow in the portal vein and hepatic artery (arrow). Seven days after transplant (right): There is hepatofugal flow in the portal vein. Increased slow flow sensitivity Doppler signal explains the lighter color hue in both arteries and veins. Pathology demonstrated severe rejection with centrilobular necrosis and periportal inflammation

HEPATOCELLULAR CARCINOMA

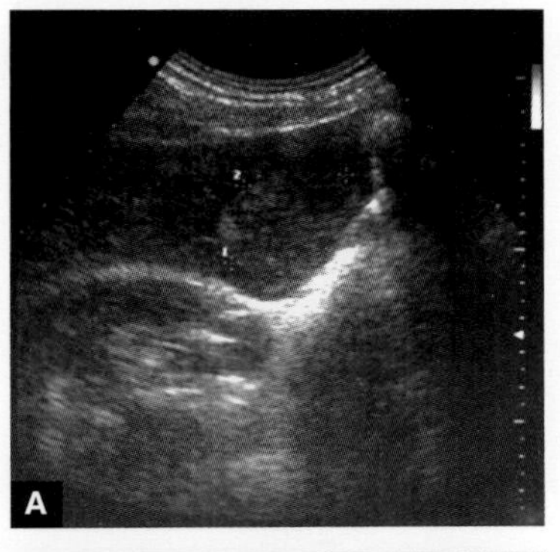

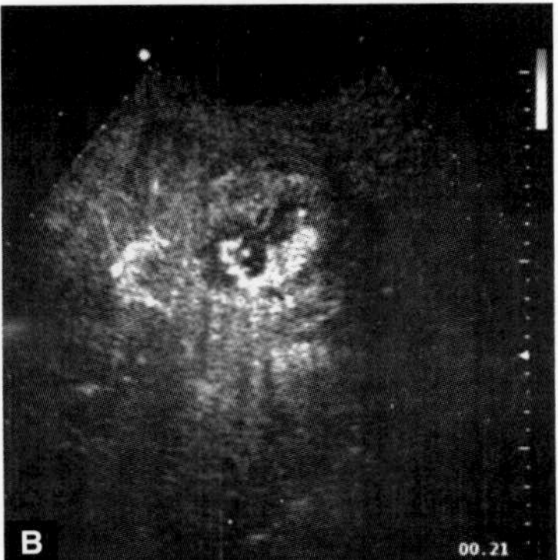

FIGURES 3.23A and B

(A) Gray scale image shows a well-defined mixed echogenicity mass lesion in the liver (B) Early arterial phase image of the lesion after contrast administration shows peripheral enhancement

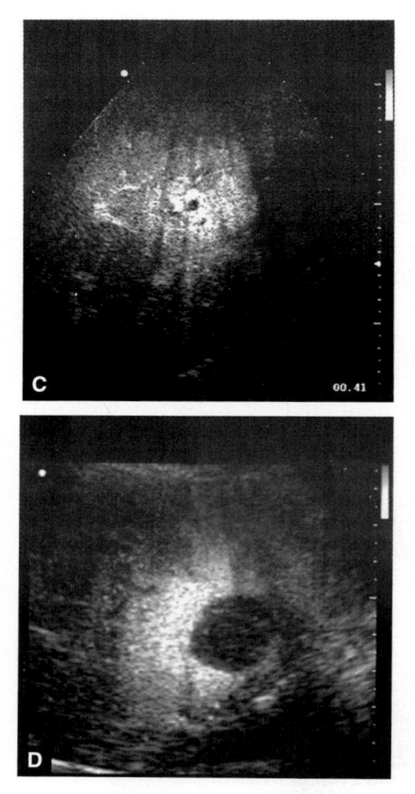

FIGURES 3.23C and D

(C) Progressive centripetal enhancement in the lesion is evident in late arterial phase (D) In the late phase, the surrounding liver enhances more than the lesion from which contrast has been washed out, leading to increased lesional conspicuity

FOCAL NODULAR HYPERPLASIA

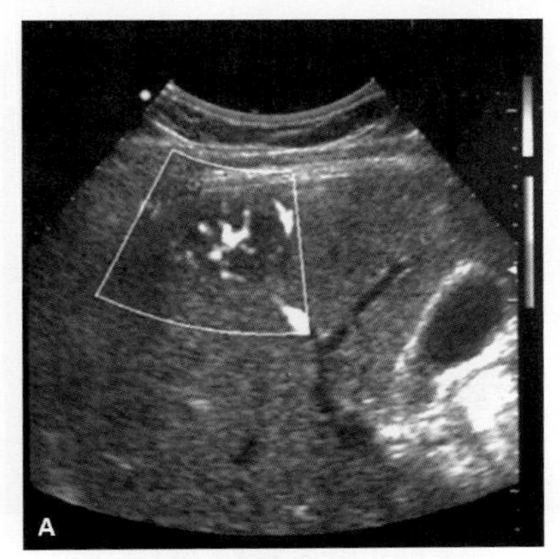

FIGURE 3.24A

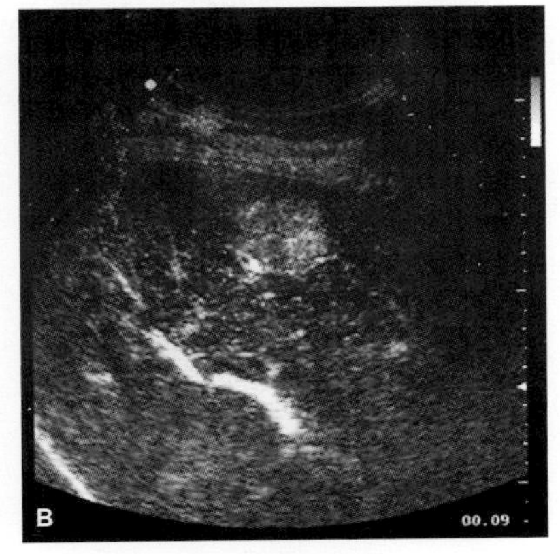

FIGURE 3.24B

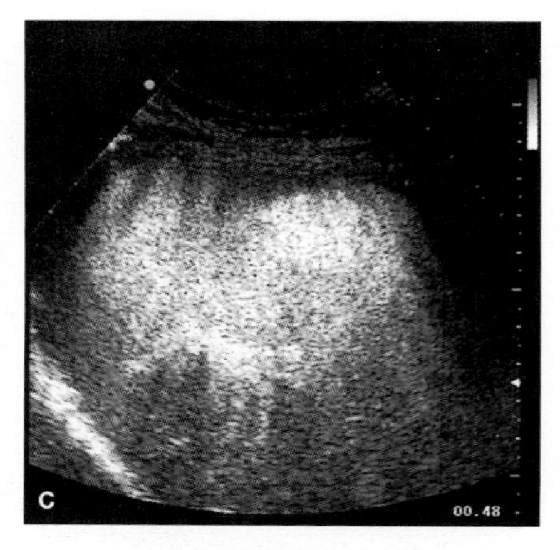

FIGURES 3.24A to C

(A) Increased vascularity is evident on power Doppler imaging, (B) Increased vascularity is also seen in early arterial phase, after contrast administration. A branch of right hepatic artery is also well visualized, (C) Late arterial phase image shows progressive contrast enhancement

Vascular plexus in FNH emanates radially from a central artery and exhibits centrifugal flow giving rise to a "spoked wheel" pattern

FOCAL LESION IN LIVER

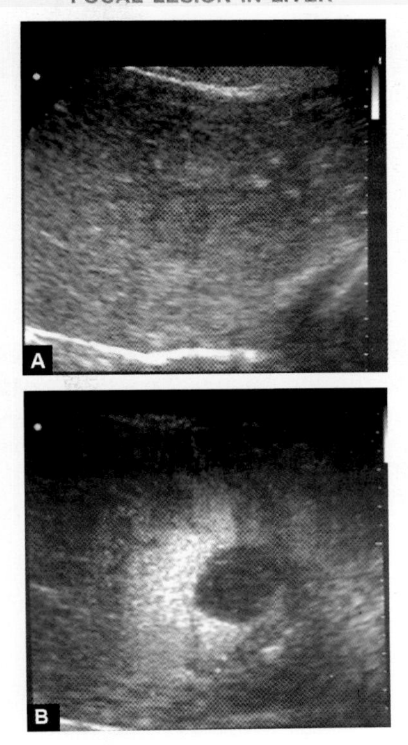

FIGURES 3.25A and B

(A) A baseline sonogram shows an ill-defined hypoechoic lesion in the liver, (B) Following contrast administration, lesion appears as a more conspicuous parenchymal defect; thus demonstrating the role of ultrasound contrast agent in detecting subtle lesions

Checklist: Portal hypertension

Suggestive signs in CDS:

- Flow velocity decreased to < 10 cm/s
- Thrombosis
- Cavernous transformation of the PV

Definite signs in CDS:

- Portocaval anastomoses
- Flow away from the liver

Rule of thumb for the differential diagnosis of hepatic lesions

Lesions that show more prolonged signal enhancement after the use of contrast agents are more likely to be benign, while metastasis and HCC often appear hypoechoic to the surrounding liver parenchyma even in the late venous phase

Chapter Four

Color Doppler in Spleen

CDI IN SPLENOMEGALY

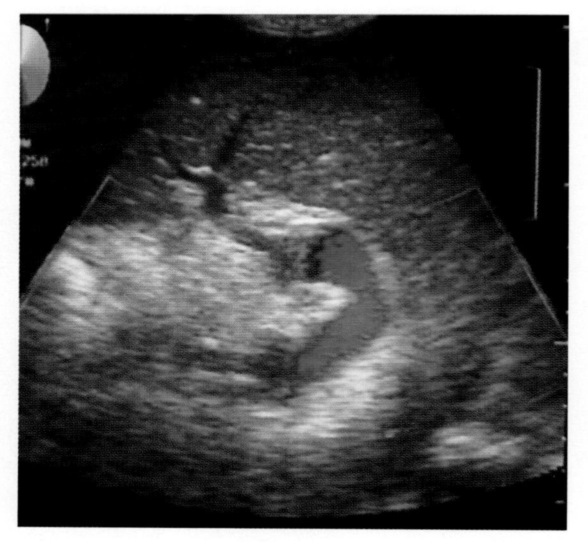

FIGURE 4.1

Color Doppler image at the splenic hilum shows dilated and tortuous splenic vein with hepatopetal blood flow in a case of splenomegaly

DDI IN PORTAL HYPERTENSION

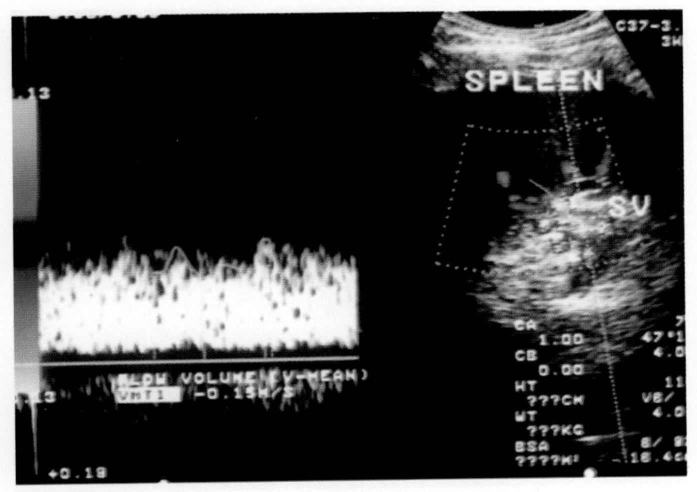

FIGURE 4.2

Duplex Doppler image shows continuous monophasic hepatopetal splenic venous flow with minimal respiratory phasicity in a case of early portal hypertension

CDI IN PORTAL HYPERTENSION

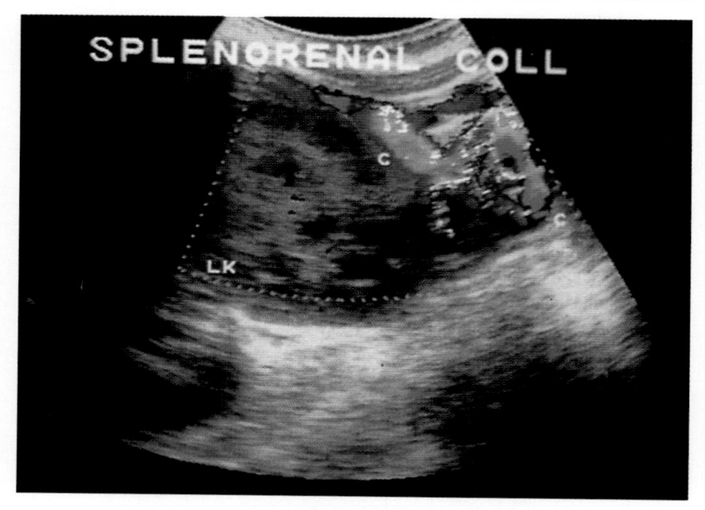

FIGURE 4.3

Color Doppler image shows multiple dilated and tortuous splenorenal (lienorenal) collaterals in a case of portal hypertension

MASS IN SPLEEN

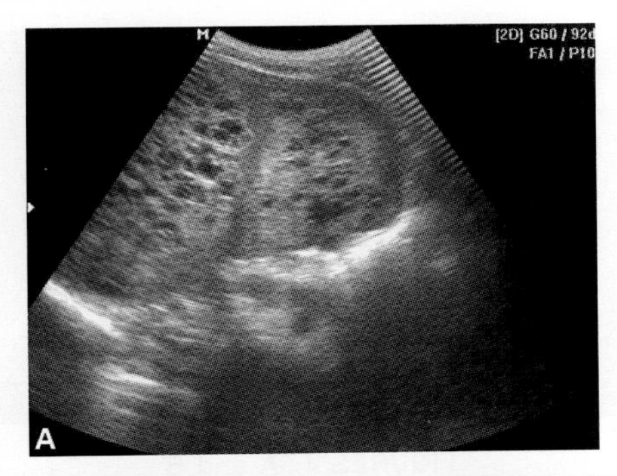

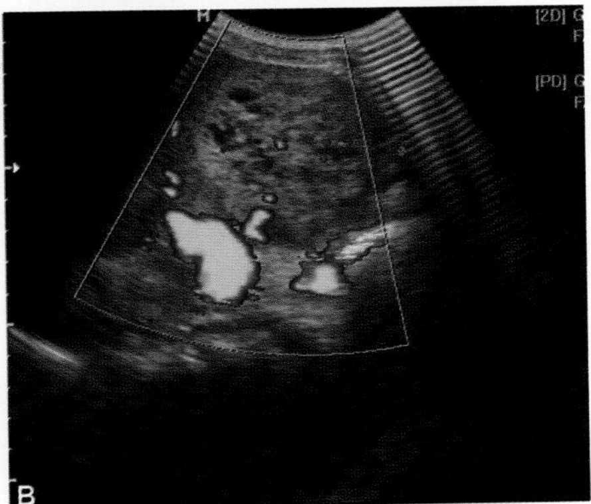

FIGURES 4.4A and B

(A) Gray scale image shows an echogenic mass with multiple tiny cystic spaces in the splenic parenchyma, (B) Power Doppler image shows minimal vascularity in the above mass; splenic vessels can be seen at the hilum

SPLENIC ARTERY ANEURYSM

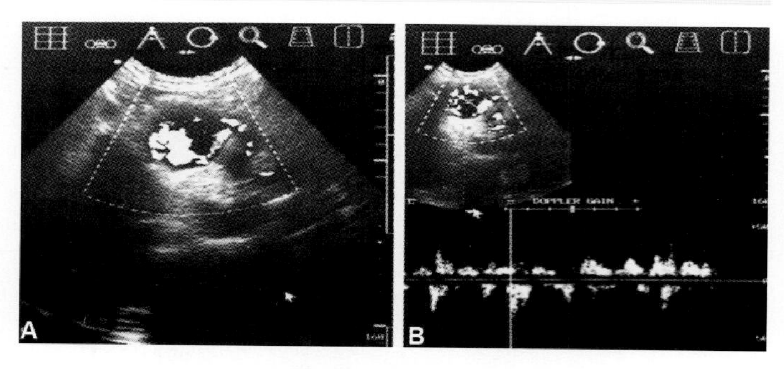

FIGURES 4.5A and B

(A) Color Doppler image shows an anechoic structure with color flow arising from the splenic artery, (B) Duplex Doppler image shows presence of both antegrade and retrograde flow with flow gradients known as to and fro motion characteristic of aneurysm

Chapter Five

Color Doppler in Urinary System

CDI IN NORMAL KIDNEY

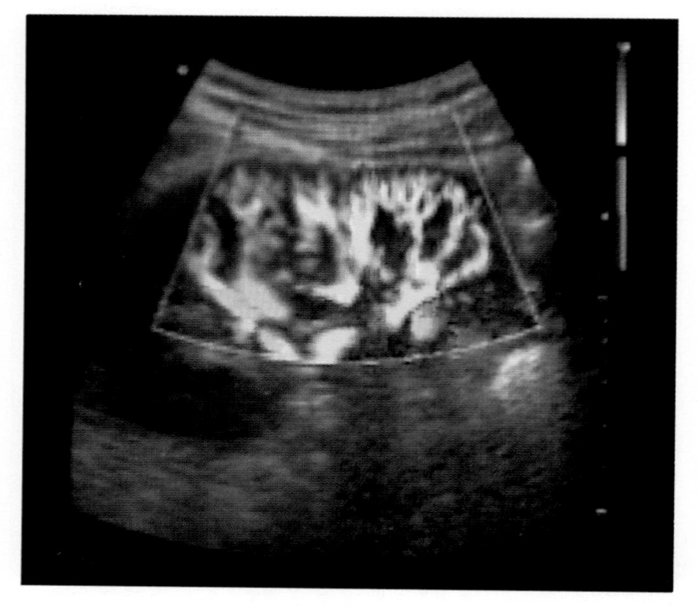

FIGURE 5.1

Color Doppler image of normal kidney at lowest PRF settings demonstrates normal appearance of intraparenchymal renal arteries and veins

POWER DOPPLER IN NORMAL KIDNEY

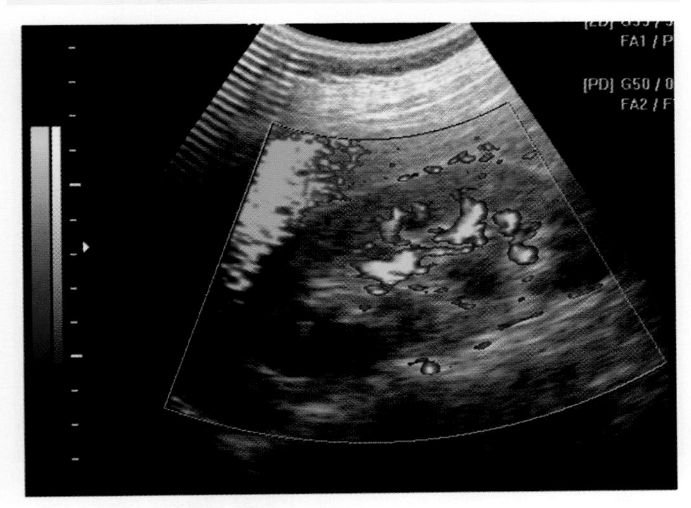

FIGURE 5.2

Power Doppler image of normal kidney at high PRF settings to visualize the vessels only at the renal hilum; blood flow is coded yellow on this color map and it can not differentiate between the arteries and veins as there is lack of directional information

DDI OF NORMAL RENAL ARTERY

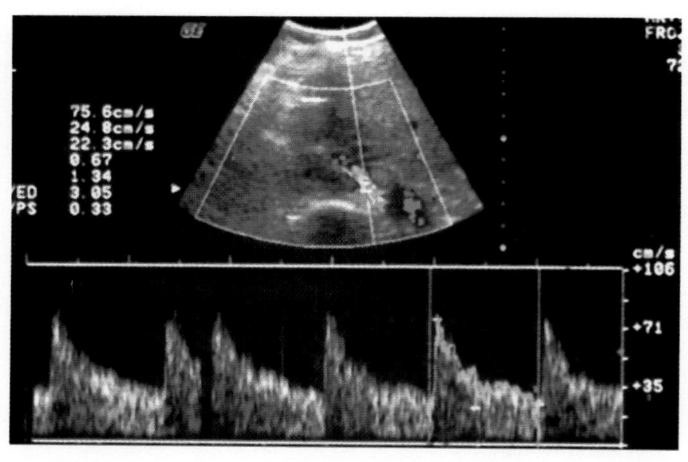

FIGURE 5.3

Duplex Doppler image of normal renal artery near the origin from aorta showing low impedance pattern with continuous forward diastolic flow

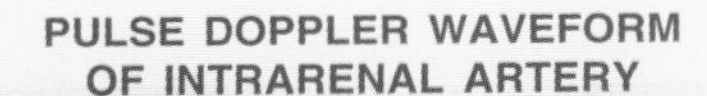

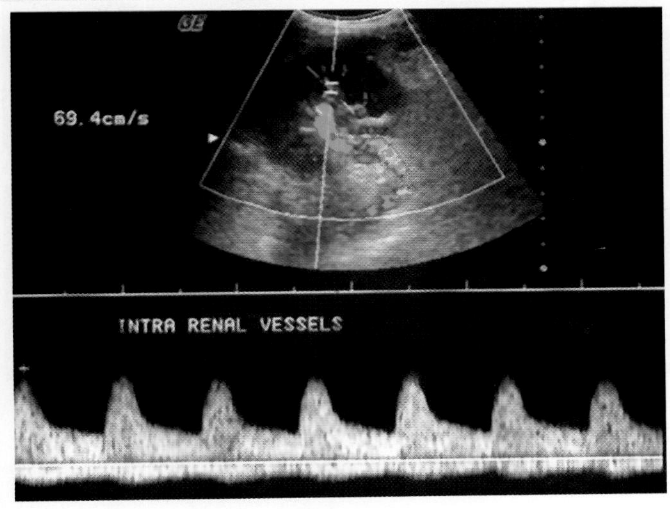

FIGURE 5.4

Normal pulse Doppler waveform of intrarenal artery shows low resistance pattern with continuous forward diastolic flow. Continuous low velocity flow seen on the other side of baseline is due to simultaneous sampling from the adjacent vein

WILMS' TUMOR

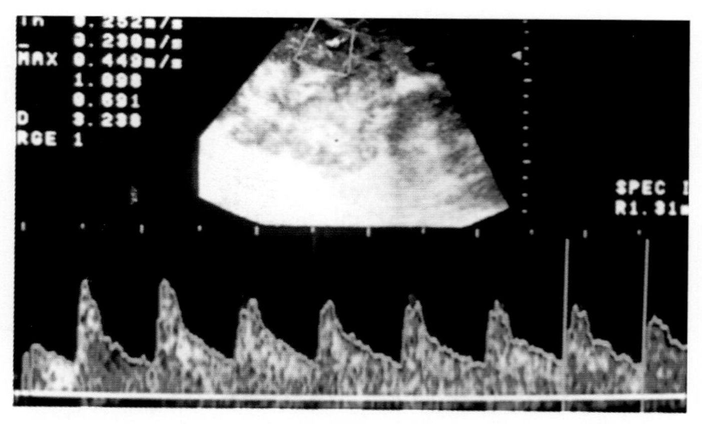

FIGURE 5.5

Duplex Doppler showing high velocity flow signals with high end diastolic velocity in a case of Wilms' tumor suggestive of a highly vascular tumor

RENAL CELL CARCINOMA

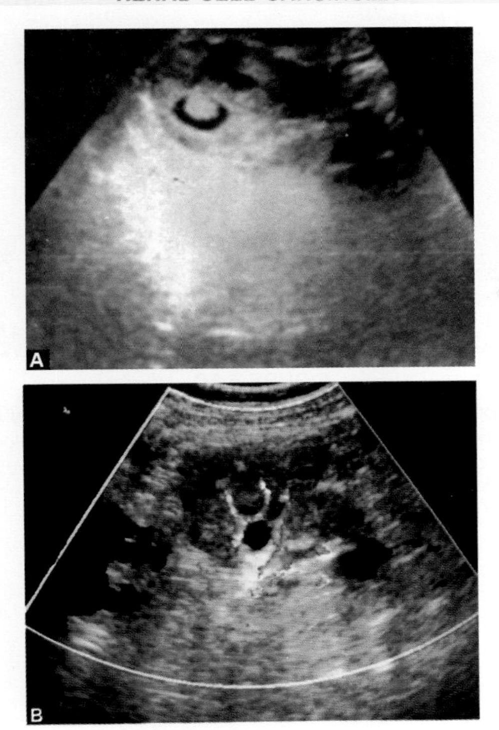

FIGURES 5.6A and B

(A) Gray scale image shows a well-defined heterogeneous mass with cystic areas (B) Color Doppler image shows moderate vascularity within the mass

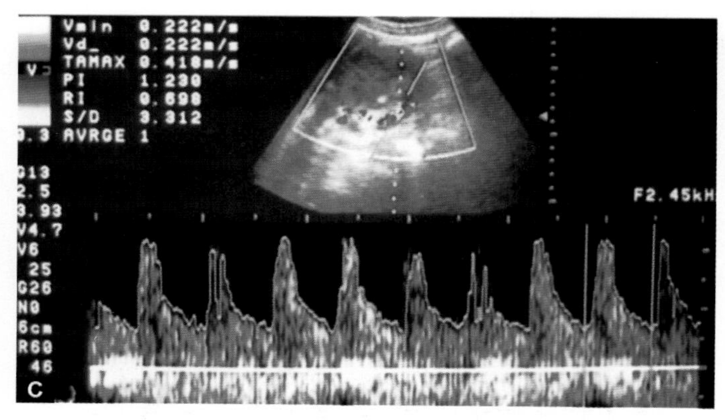

FIGURE 5.6C

Duplex Doppler image in another patient shows high velocity and low resistance waveform characterized by high peak systolic velocity and continuous diastolic flow

PLAQUE IN A CASE OF RENAL HYPERTENSION

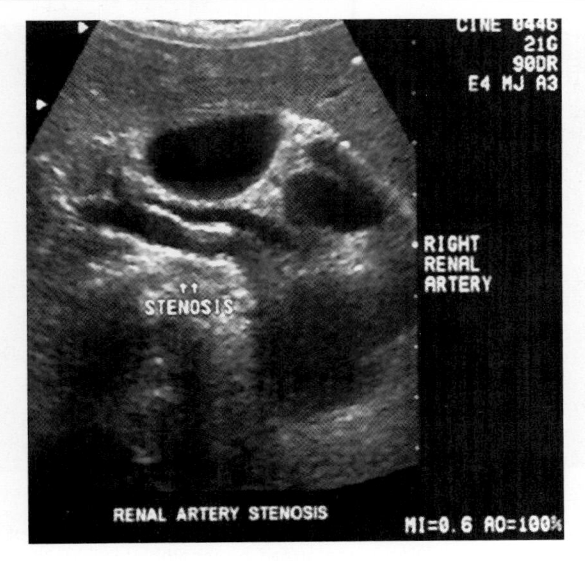

FIGURE 5.7

Gray scale image shows a plaque at the origin of right renal artery causing significant luminal narrowing in a patient with renal hypertension

CDI IN RENAL HYPERTENSION

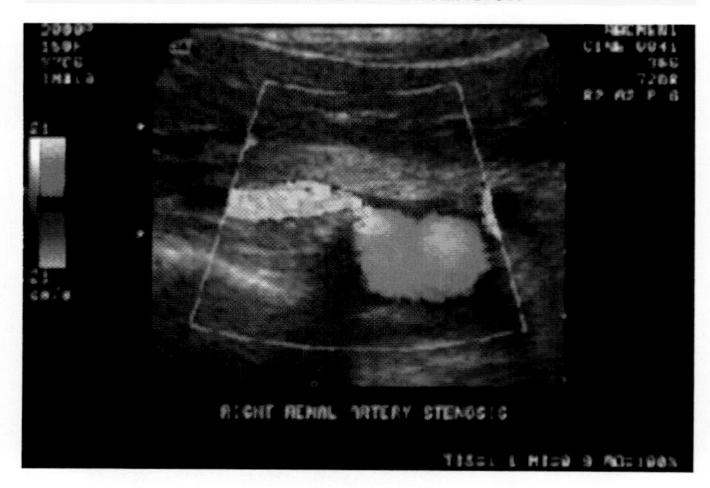

FIGURE 5.8

Color Doppler flow image in another patient showing narrowing of right renal artery at its origin characterized by incomplete color filling the lumen

PULSE DOPPLER IN RENAL ARTERY STENOSIS

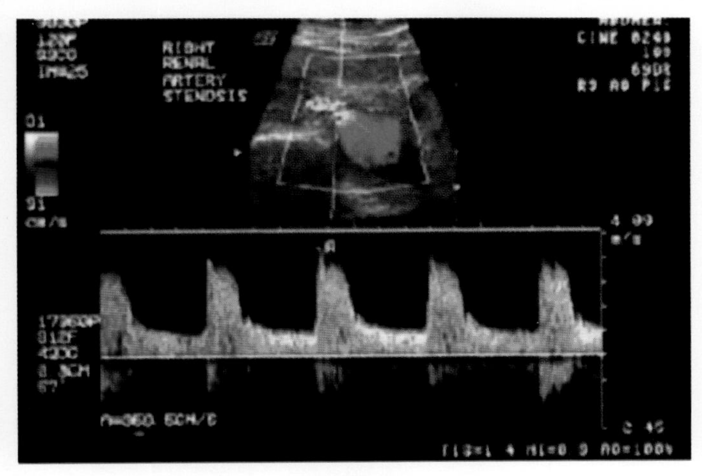

FIGURE 5.9

Pulse Doppler tracing at the point of narrowing shows high peak systolic velocity in renal artery with filling of the systolic window suggestive of turbulence

WAVEFORM IN RAS

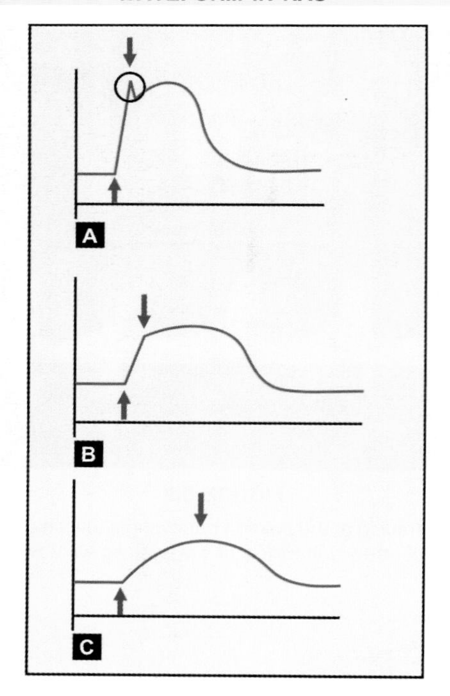

FIGURES 5.10A to C

Schematic representation of the renal artery waveform in renal artery stenosis:, (A) 0 to 59 per cent RAS (B) 60 to 79 per cent RAS, (C) 80 or more per cent RAS. Note: Top arrow: early systolic peak (ESP) and Bottom arrow: beginning of early systolic

ENLARGED, HETEROECHOIC RT KIDNEY

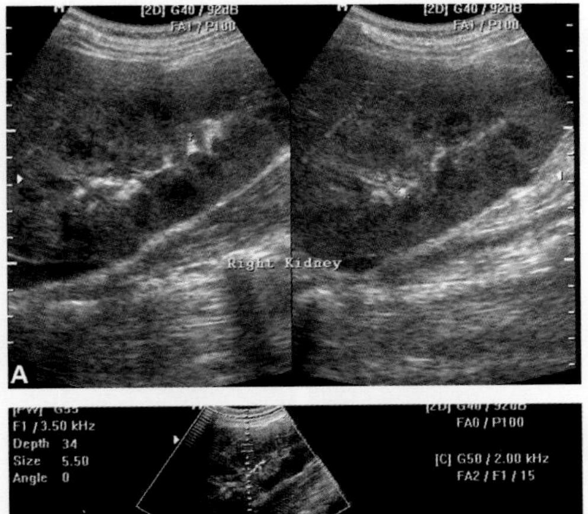

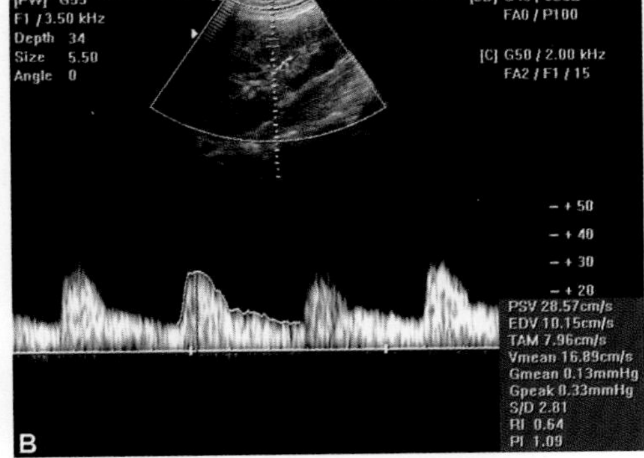

FIGURES 5.11A and B

(A) Gray scale image shows enlarged and heteroechoic right kidney with perinephric collection near the upper pole and a small upper pole calculus, (B) Duplex Doppler image shows high RI value in the intrarenal vessel of the same kidney suggestive of altered renal perfusion

RENAL TRANSPLANT REJECTION

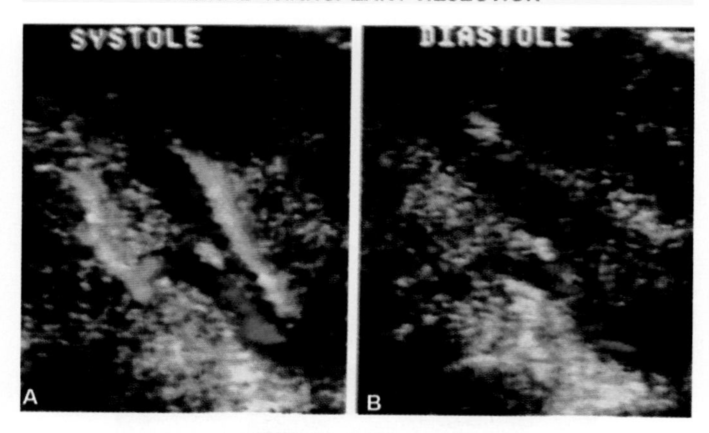

FIGURES 5.12A and B

Color Doppler showing a forward flow during systole (A) while no flow in diastole (B) which is characteristic of moderate or high impedance pattern

TRANSPLANT REJECTION KIDNEY

These findings are suggestive of transplant rejection at both interstitial and vascular level

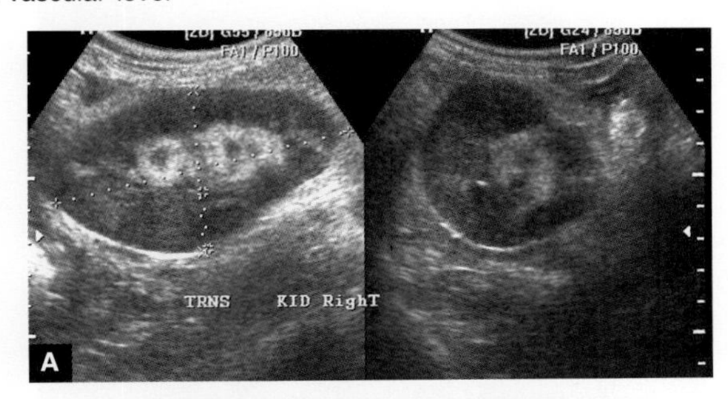

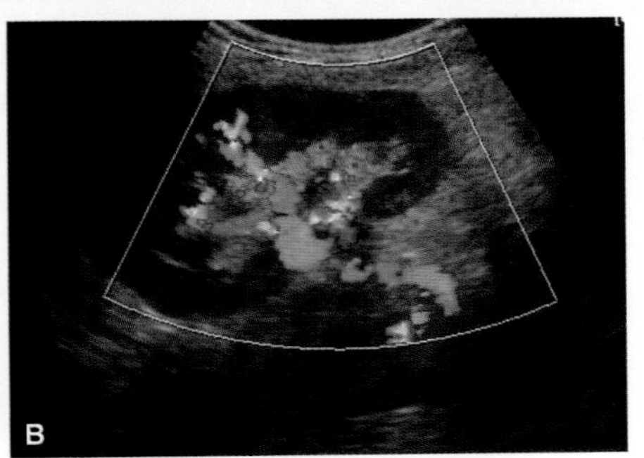

FIGURES 5.13A and B

(A) B-mode image shows a hypoechoic transplanted kidney with loss of corticomedullary differentiation (B) Color Doppler image with minimum PRF settings shows flow in the main renal vessels and midpolar region but relative absence of flow at the poles

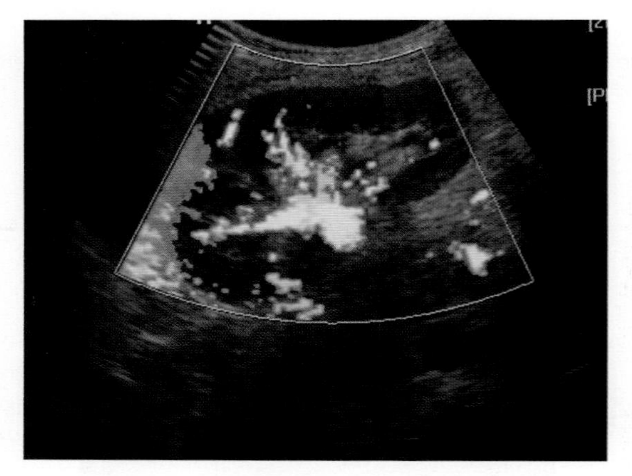

FIGURE 5.13C

Power Doppler image with minimum PRF settings shows major flow into the medulla in the midpolar region

JET FLOW IN CDI

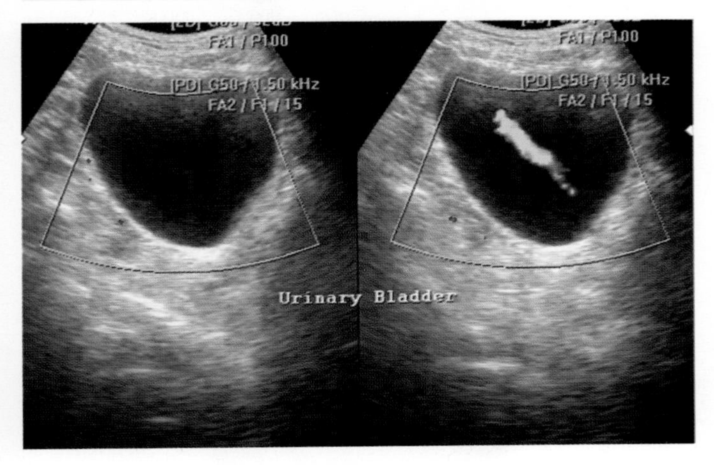

FIGURE 5.14

Gray scale image on left with color Doppler mode and on right with power Doppler image shows color flow produced by normal jet of urine in the urinary bladders. This also shows the high sensitivity of power Doppler in detecting flow

VUR

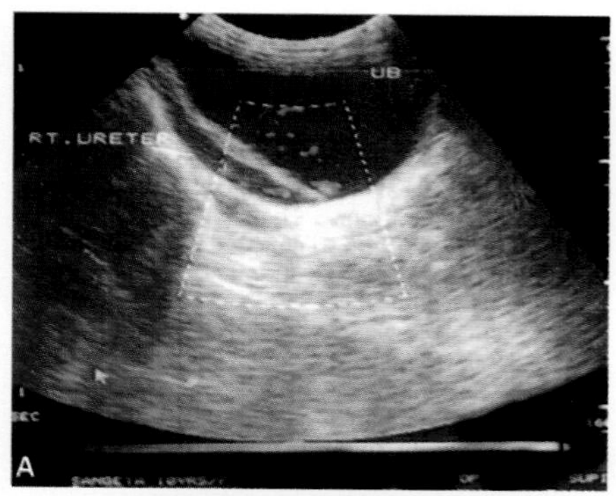

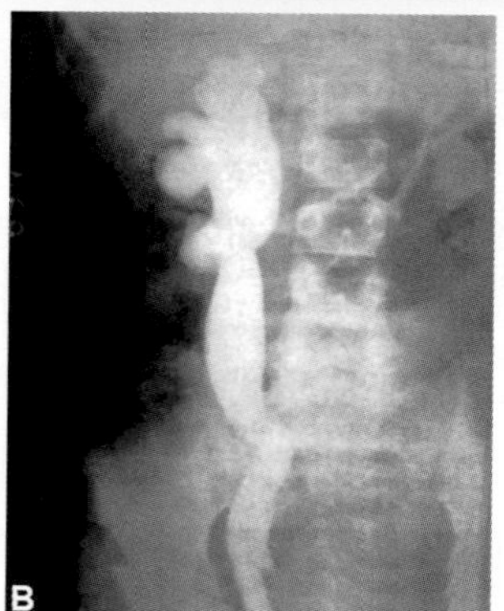

FIGURES 5.15A and B

(A) Sagittal scan color Doppler image shows dilated right lower ureter with VUR seen as blue color, (B) Voiding cystourethrogram of the same patient showing Grade V reflux

MASS IN URINARY BLADDER

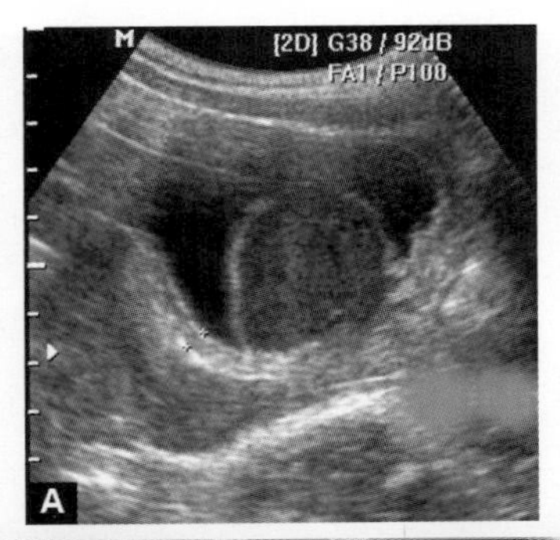

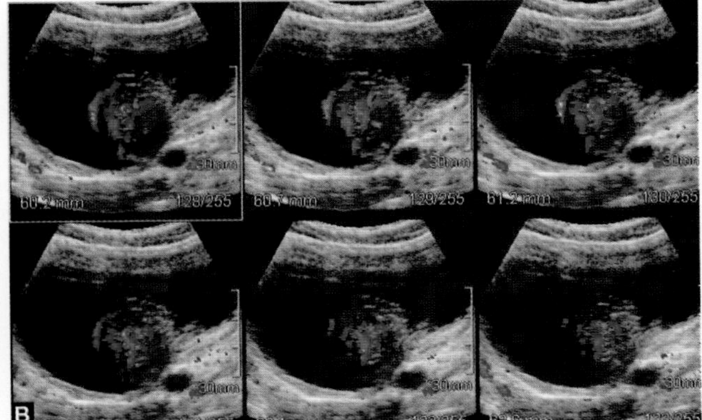

FIGURES 5.16A and B

(A) Gray scale image shows a hypoechoic mass within the urinary bladder, (B) Multiple axial 3D-Color Doppler images reveal high vascularity within the lesion suggesting a hemangioma (biopsy proved)

PROSTATE MALIGNANCY

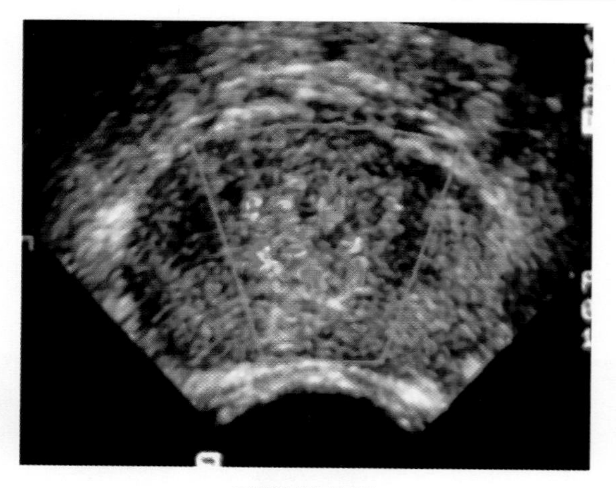

FIGURE 5.17

Color Doppler image of prostate obtained through transrectal US shows focal hypoechoic lesion with increased vascularity and haphazard vessels characteristic of malignant lesion

Normal RI values in the interlobar artries of hypertensive patients		
Age (years)	*m*	*m + 2 SD*
<20	0.567	0.523-0.611
21-30	0.573	0.528-0.618
31-40	0.588	0.546-0.630
41-50	0.618	0.561-0.675
51-60	0.668	0.603-0.733
61-70	0.732	0.649-0.815
71-80	0.781	0.707-0.855
>81	0.832	

Renal artery stenosis can be labelled if
1. Acceleration time > 70 ms (measured in the segmental arteries)
2. PSV > 200 cm/s (Direct criteria)
3. RI on each side is below the age normal range—Bilateral RAS (Indirect criteria)
Rt - Lt. difference in RI Values > 0.05 (Indirect criteria)

CDS is indicated in
1. Hypertension in a patient under 30 years of age
2. Creatinine rise while on treatment with ACE inhibitors or AT –1 receptor antagonists
3. Diastolic blood pressure > 105 mm Hg despite triple antihypertensive regimen, especially in patients with severe generalized atherosclerosis
4. More than 1.5 cm right-left discrepancy in renal size.

Chapter Six

Color Doppler in Retroperitoneum and Great Vessels

TIME VELOCITY SPECTRA

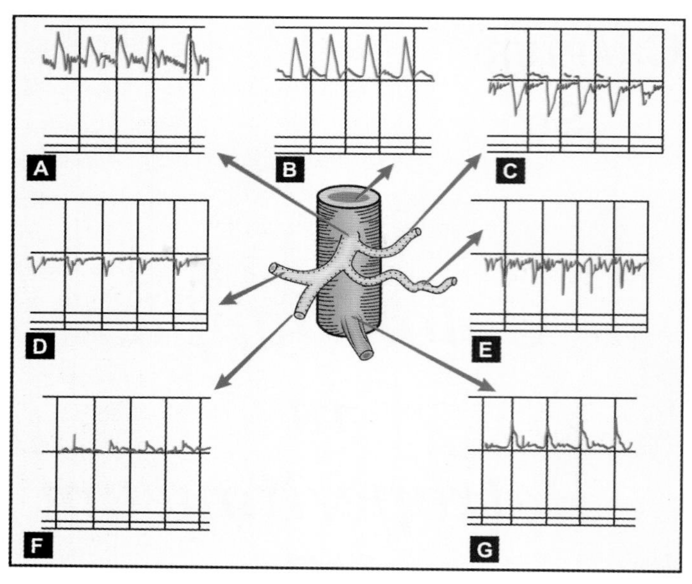

FIGURE 6.1

In celiac trunk (A), proximal aorta (B), left gastric artery (C), common hepatic artery (D), splenic artery (E), gastroduodenal artery (F), and superior mesenteric artery (G)

TIME VELOCITY SPECTRA

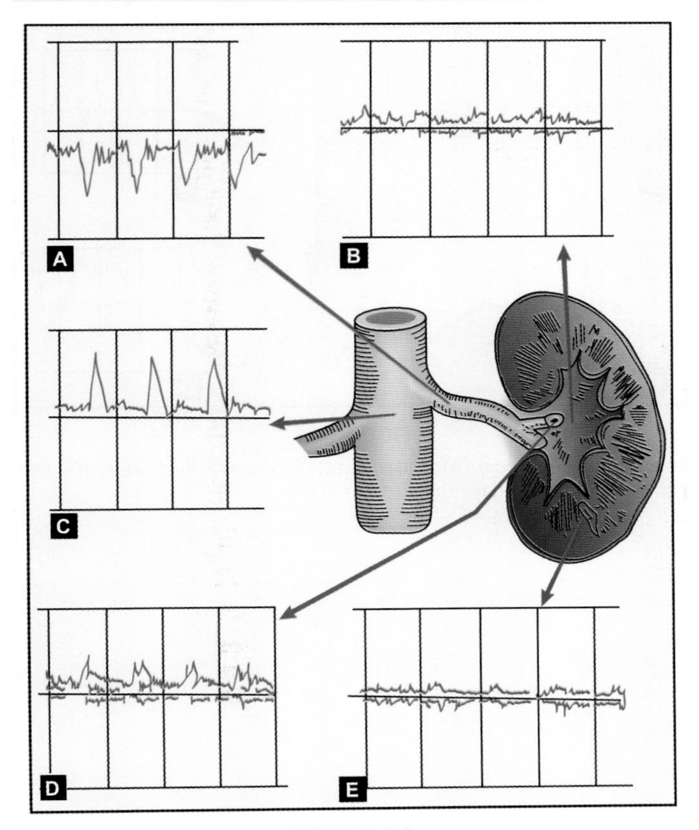

FIGURE 6.2

In main renal artery at origin (A); mid zone of kidney (B); mid-aorta (C); renal sinus (D); arcuate artery (E)

TIME VELOCITY SPECTRA

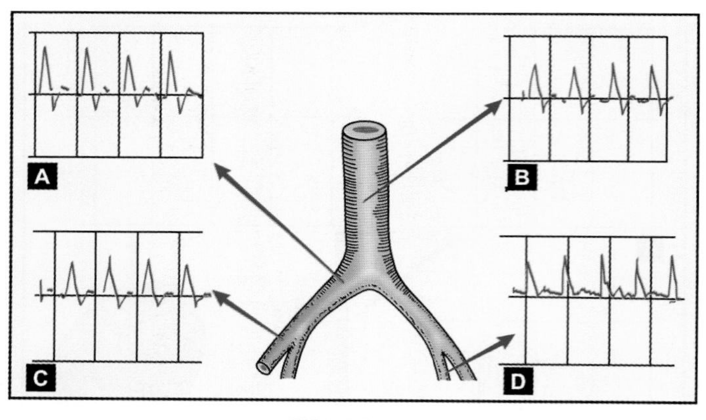

FIGURE 6.3

In common iliac artery (A), distal aorta, (B) external iliac artery (C) and internal iliac artery (D)

ATHEROSCLEROTIC PLAQUE IN ABDOMINAL AORTA

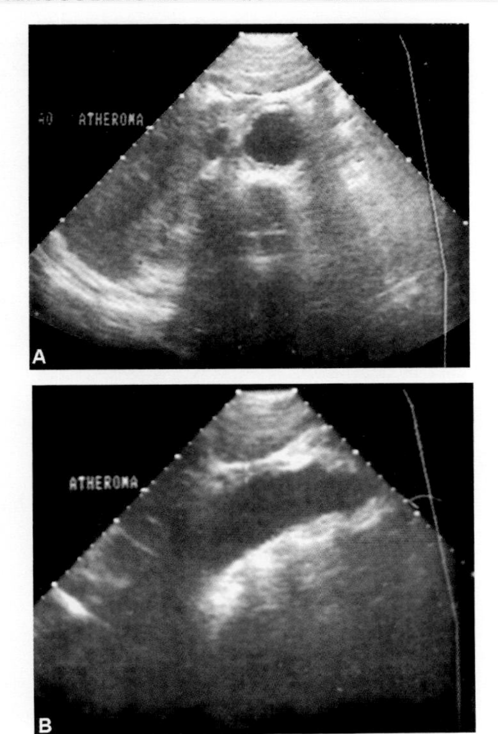

FIGURES 6.4A and B

Gray scale images show dilated abdominal aorta with atherosclerotic plaque in transverse scan (A), and longitudinal scan (B). Presence of echogenicity within the plaque suggests calcification

THROMBUS IN AORTA

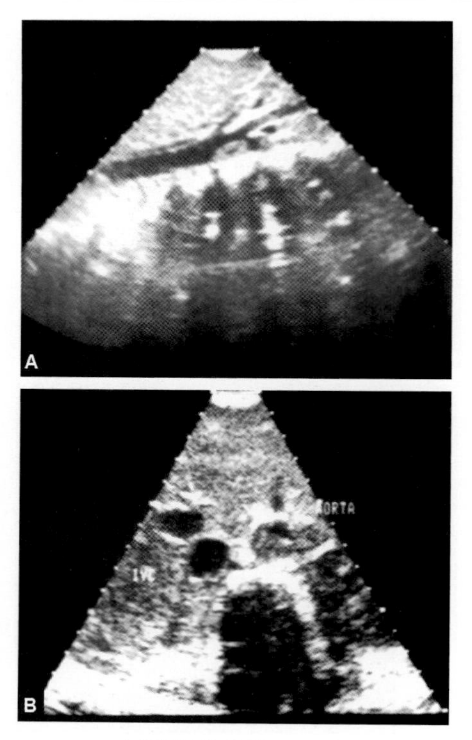

FIGURES 6.5A and B

Gray scale images show thrombus in the lumen of aorta along the posterior wall at the level of origin of superior mesenteric artery from aorta as seen on (A) longitudinal scan and (B) transverse scan. The origin of superior mesenteric artery is not affected but velocity pattern will be altered resulting in SMA syndrome like symptoms

AORTIC PSEUDOANEURYSM WITH THROMBUS

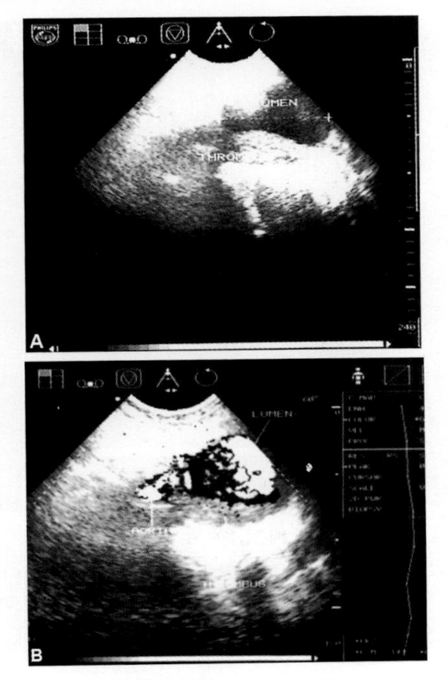

FIGURES 6.6A and B

(A) Gray scale image in transverse plane at mid-aortic level showing well defined, anechoic saccular outpouching from the aorta. An echogenic thrombus is seen along the posterior wall (aortic pseudoaneurysm), (B) Color flow Doppler image of same patient shows variable color flow pattern in the lumen characteristic of pseudoaneurysm

DUPLEX DOPPLER IN NORMAL IVC

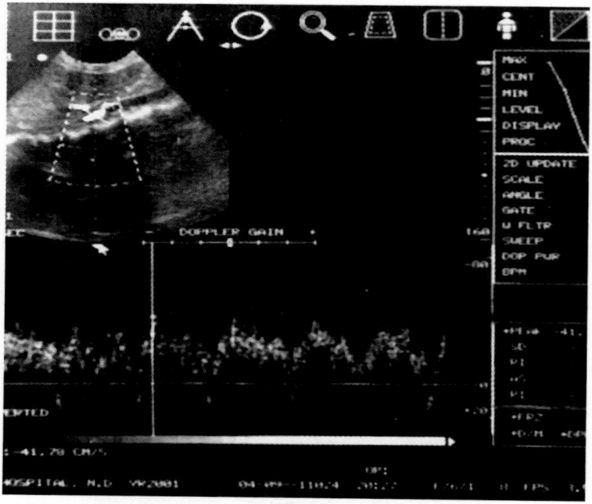

FIGURE 6.7

Duplex Doppler of normal IVC showing wide variation in flow velocity and direction owing to effects of cardiac and respiratory cycles

THROMBUS IN IVC

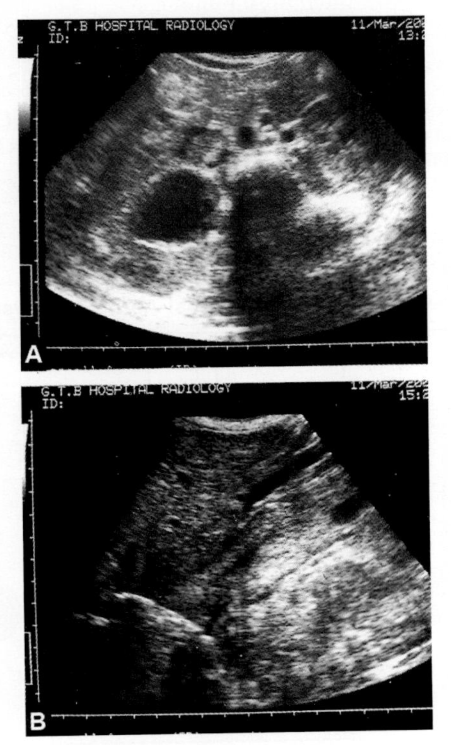

FIGURES 6.8A and B

Gray scale image in transverse (A) and longitudinal sections (B) showing an echogenic thrombus partially obliterating the lumen of inferior vena cava and extending along its length. Such thrombus has a high propensity to produce pulmonary thromboembolism

Criteria for aortic dilatation	
1.	Flow laminar or turbulent
2.	Max, AO diameter: < 2.5 cm Indication for surgery: > 5 cm, progression of >0.5 cm/year
3.	Width and location of perfused, thrombozed or false lumen: eccentric location.
4.	Involvement of renal, visceral, or iliac arteries? (surgical strategy and implant selection)
5.	Peripheral aneurysmosis?
6.	Spectra in true and false lumen? (impending ischemia, indication for surgery)

Classification of Abdominal Aortic Aneurysm

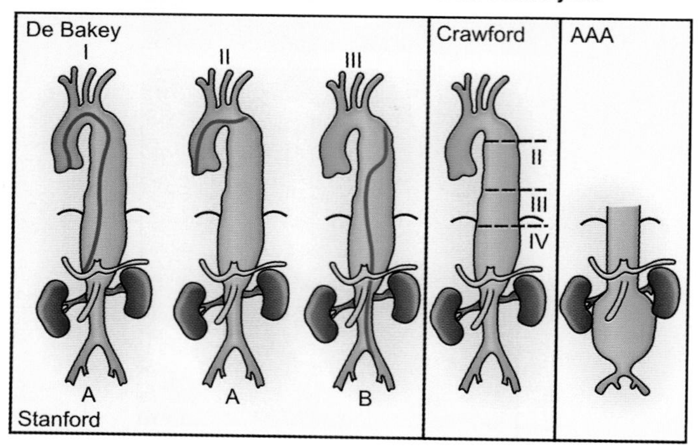

Risk of rupture when-

1. Flow is turbulent
2. Maximum AO diameter > 7.5 cm
3. When location is eccentric

Chapter Seven

Color Doppler in Scrotal and Penile Pathologies

DDI IN INTRATESTICULAR ARTERY

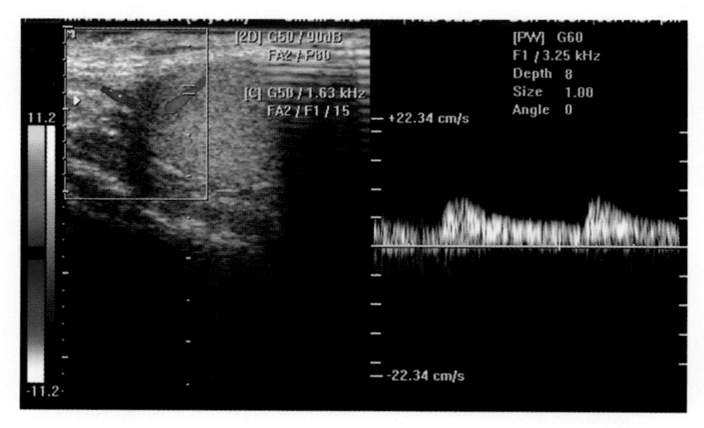

FIGURE 7.1

Duplex Doppler image shows low velocity and low resistance flow i.e. low impedance flow in the intratesticular artery characteristic of end arteries

POWER DOPPLER – NORMAL TESTICULAR VASCULARITY

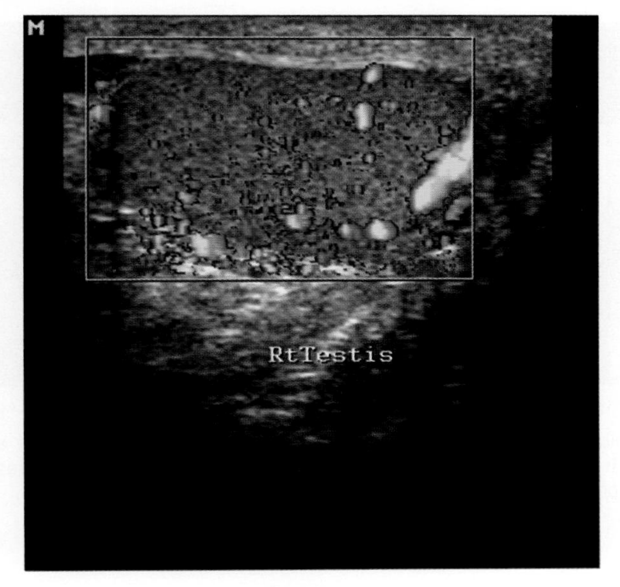

FIGURE 7.2

Power Doppler shows normal pattern of testicular vascularity with major vascularity seen in the region of mediastinum testis

COLOR DOPPLER—NORMAL PAMPINIFORM PLEXUS

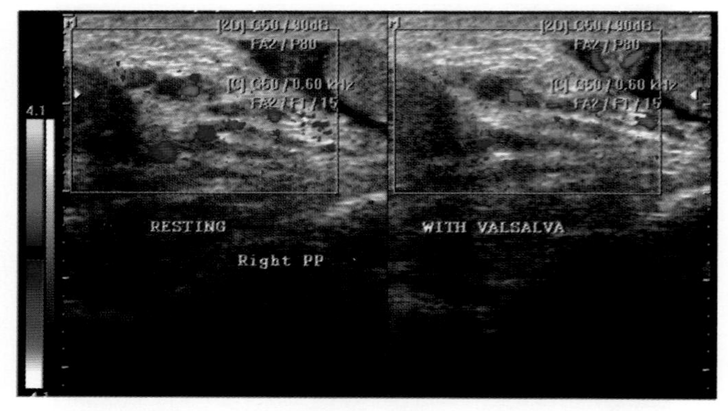

FIGURE 7.3

Color Doppler shows normal pampiniform plexus in resting state and with Valsalva maneuver. Notice there is no dilatation of veins, no increase in color and no reversal of color

TORSION OF TESTIS

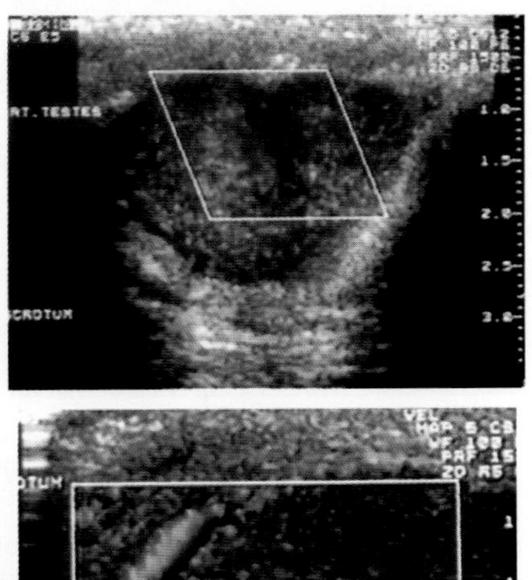

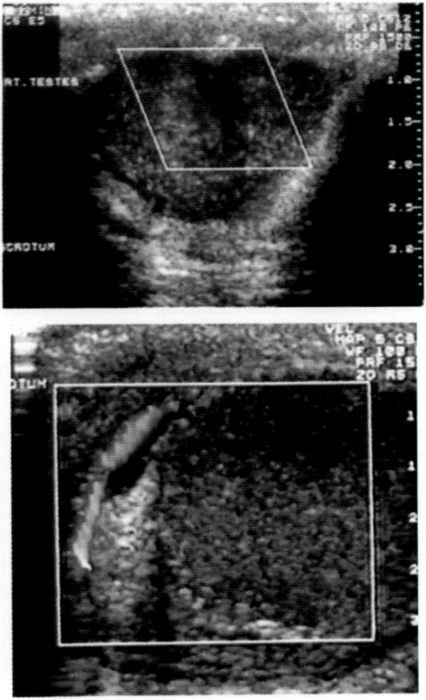

FIGURES 7.4A and B

(A) Complete absence of color flow in the testis at lowest PRF settings. Late phase of testicular torsion (B) Color Doppler image shows no flow is seen in the testis but flow is seen in the testicular artery prior to the site of torsion

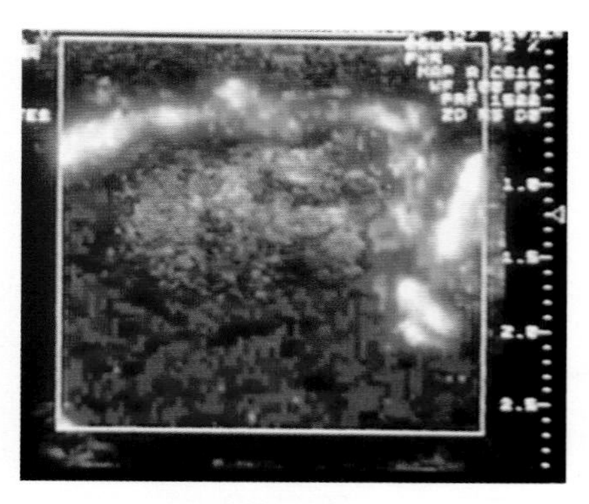

FIGURE 7.4C

Power Doppler highlights exuberant peri-testicular flow and absence of flow in the testis

Always remember—The most sonographically detectable change in initial hours after testicular torsion is absent or decreased perfusion of symptomatic side compared to opposite side. The degree of hypoperfusion of the affected side depends on duration and severity of torsion. With subtotal torsion, some residual perfusion of the affected testis can be detected. Venous obstruction precedes arterial obstruction in less severe cases with the result arterial spectra can still be recorded on the affected side while venous not. Suspect testicular torsion and proceed for surgical intervention to avoid hemorrhagic infarction.

In B-mode it takes 6-8 hours for changes to appear. Testis enlarged, parenchyma becomes nonhomogeneous and echopenic. Scrotal skin thickened on the effected side and hydrocele develops.

FUNNICULITIS

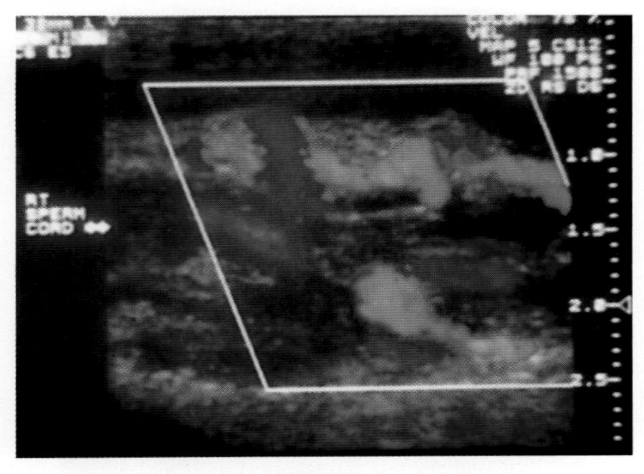

FIGURE 7.5

Color Doppler image in a case of funniculitis shows hypervascularity along the spermatic cord (post-operative infection)

ACUTE EPIDIDYMITIS

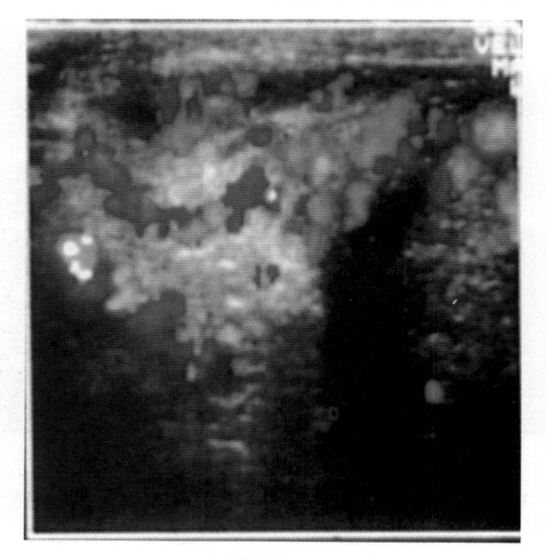

FIGURE 7.6

Color Doppler image in a case of an acute epididymitis shows hypervascularity in the form of abundant color flow in epididymis.

B mode shows enlarged epididymis with non-homogeneous internal echo pattern. Doppler spectrum shows marked increase in diastolic flow with decreased resistive index.

ACUTE ORCHITIS

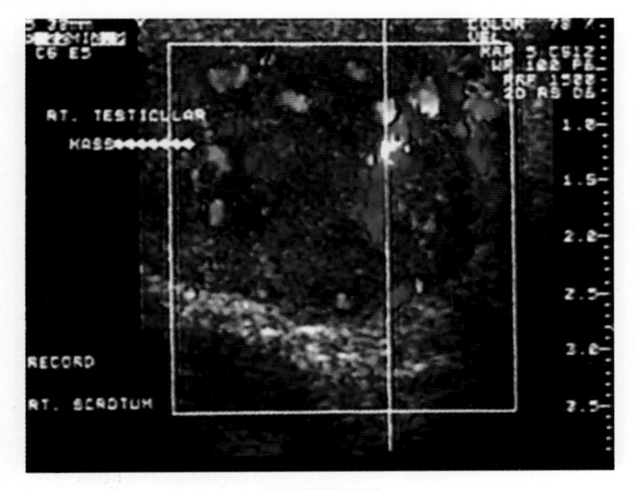

FIGURE 7.7

Color Doppler image in a case of an acute orchitis shows hypervascularity in the form of abundant color flow in testis

CHRONIC EPIDIDYMO-ORCHITIS

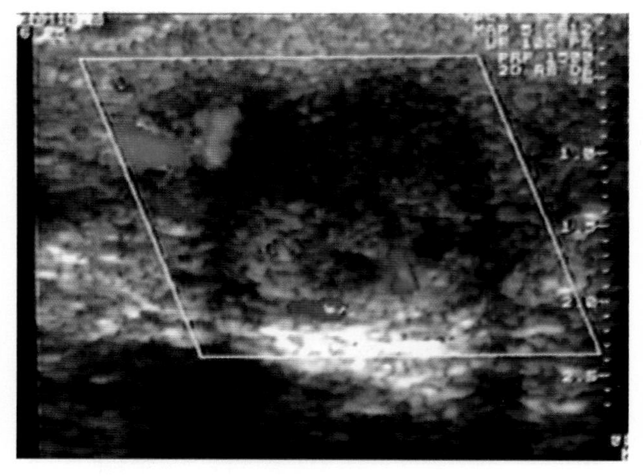

FIGURE 7.8

Color Doppler image in a case of chronic epididymo-orchitis (Tuberculous) shows small hypoechoic testis with minimal color flow. Acute inflammation is associated with enlargement of testis with increased vascularity

DILATED PAMPINIFORM PLEXUS

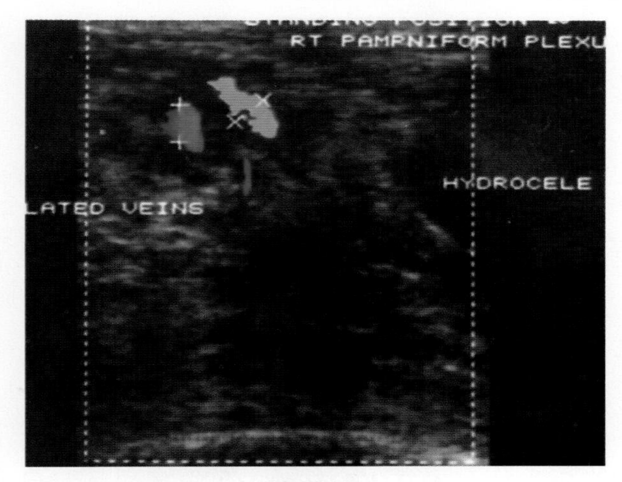

FIGURE 7.9

Color Doppler image shows dilated vein in the pampiniform plexus (diameter more than 3 mm)

VARICOCELES

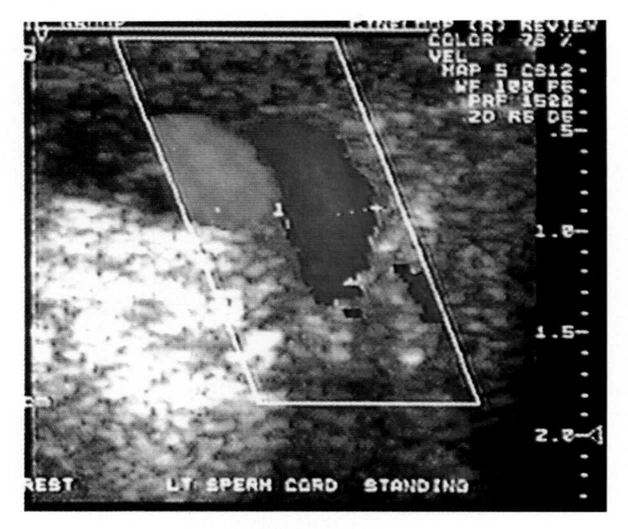

FIGURE 7.10

Longitudinal color Doppler image of the spermatic cord demonstrating dilated vascular channels suggestive of varicoceles

VARICOCELES

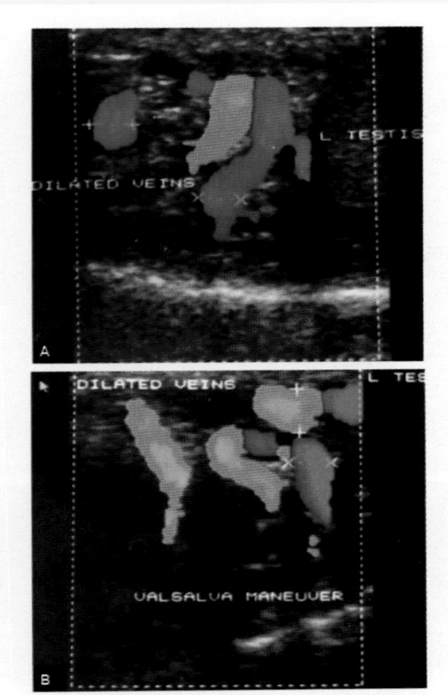

FIGURES 7.11A and B

(A) Color Doppler image shows dilated veins in standing position in a patient of varicoceles. Sometimes, varicoceles are missed, if the patient is not examined in erect posture, (B) Color Doppler shows dilated veins during Valsalva maneuver, which should always be performed even if the dilated veins are not visualized and may be the cause of hypofertility Note: The advantage of color Duplex over clinical examination alone lies in the ability of CDS to detect subclinical varicoceles. When used in regular follow-up after varicocele treatment, CDS can detect recurrence of disease at an early stage.

SEMINOMA OF TESTIS

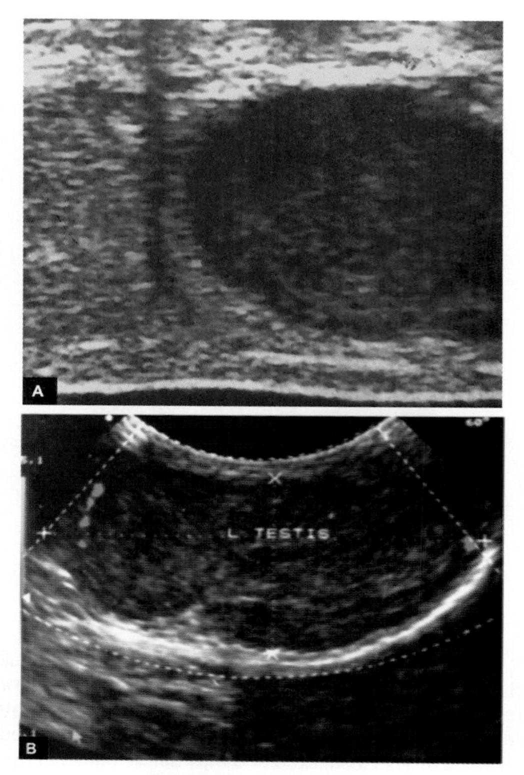

FIGURES 7.12A and B

(A) Gray scale image shows enlarged testis with uniform hypoechoic echotexture with no recognizable normal parenchyma, (B) Color Doppler image shows vascularity only at the periphery of the lesion

TERATOMA

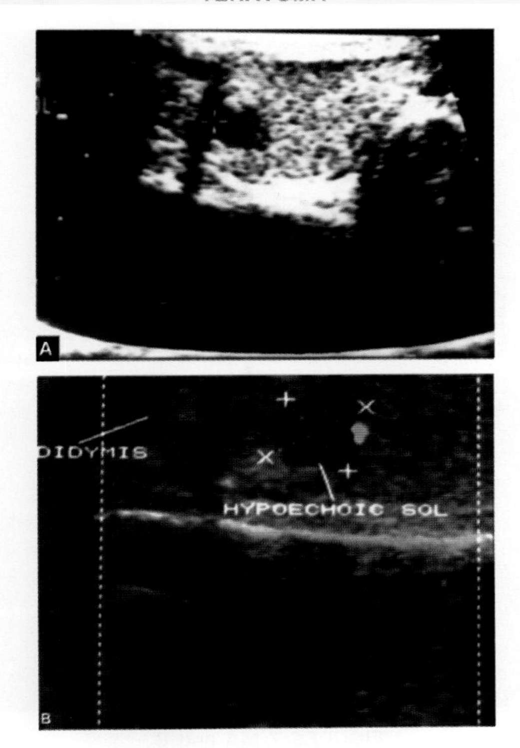

FIGURES 7.13A and B

(A) Gray scale image shows hypoechoic mass with ill-defined margins at superior pole of testis, (B) Color Doppler image shows peripheral vascularity with absence of central vascularity suggestive of relatively avascular lesion

SENILE TESTICULAR ATROPHY IN A 62-YEAR-OLD MALE

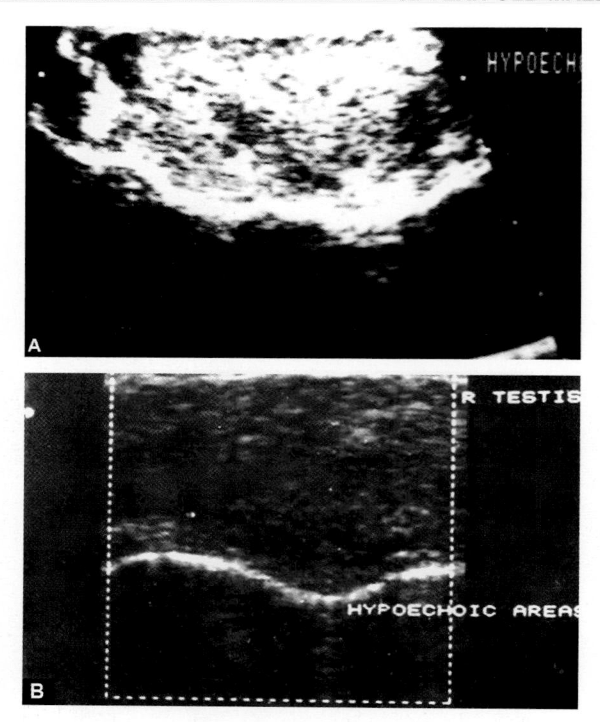

FIGURES 7.14A and B

(A) Gray scale image reveals multiple hypoechoic areas within the testis, (B) Color Doppler flow image shows avascular nature of hypoechoic areas. However, the condition has to be differentiated with granulomatous especially tubercular disease

RHABDOMYOSARCOMA SCROTUM

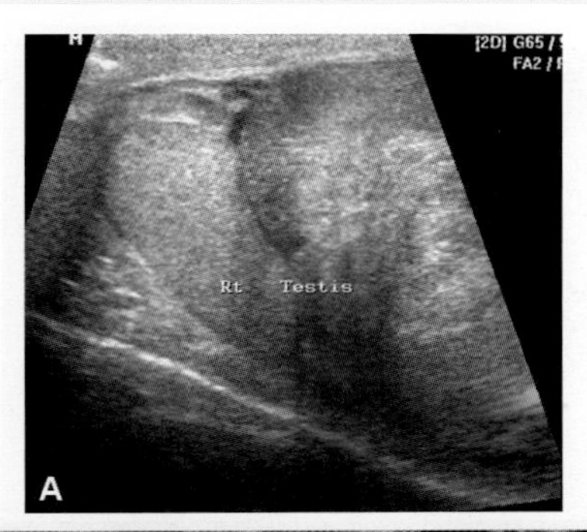

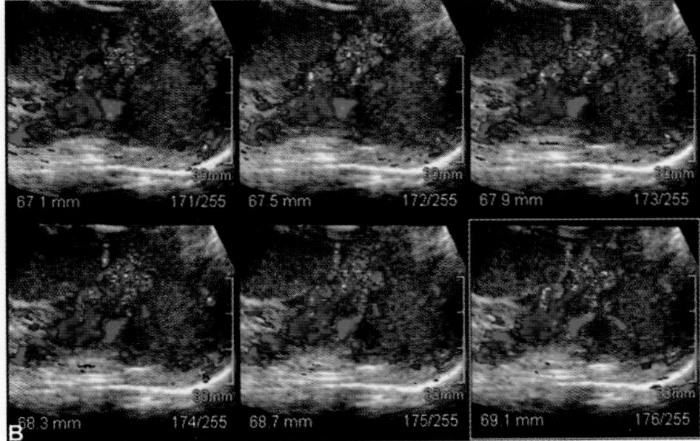

FIGURES 7.15A and B

(A) Gray scale image shows a heteroechoic solid extratesticular mass compressing the testis, (B) Multiple axial 3D Color Doppler scans reveal high and haphazard vascularity within the lesion suggestive of a sarcomatous lesion. (Proven case of rhabdomyosarcoma of scrotum)

LIPOSARCOMA

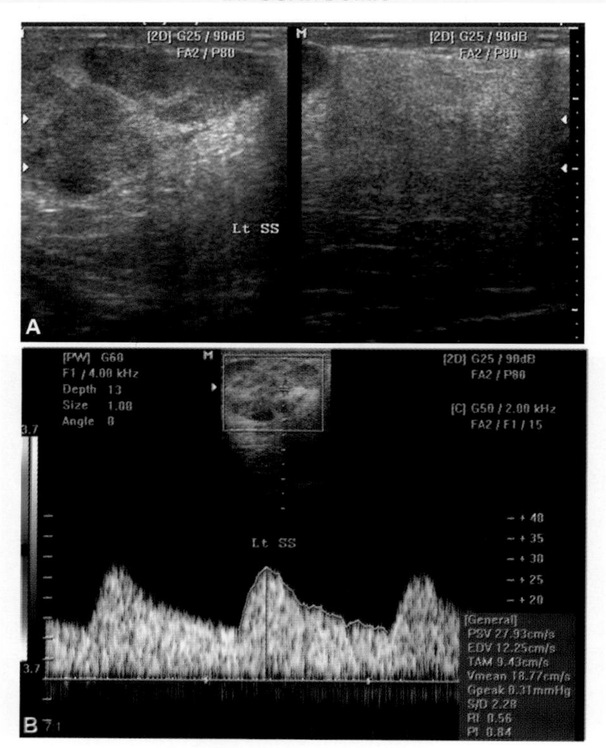

FIGURES 7.16A and B

(A) Gray scale image shows a heteroechoic predominantly echogenic mass in the scrotum suggestive of a lipomatous tumor, (B) Multiple axial 3D color Doppler scans reveal high vascularity with moderate RI and PSV suggestive of a sarcomatous lesion (biopsy was liposarcoma)

TECHNIQUE FOR SAMPLE VOLUME

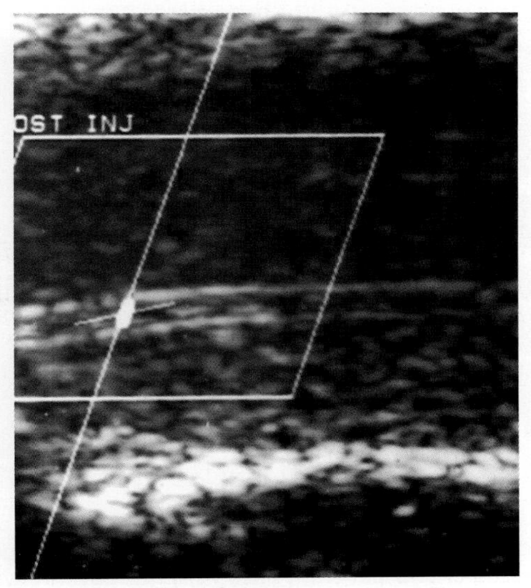

FIGURE 7.17

PPDU examination shows technique for placement of sample volume in the cavernosal artery with angle correction

FLOW PATTERN DURING POST-PAPAVERINE DOPPLER STUDY

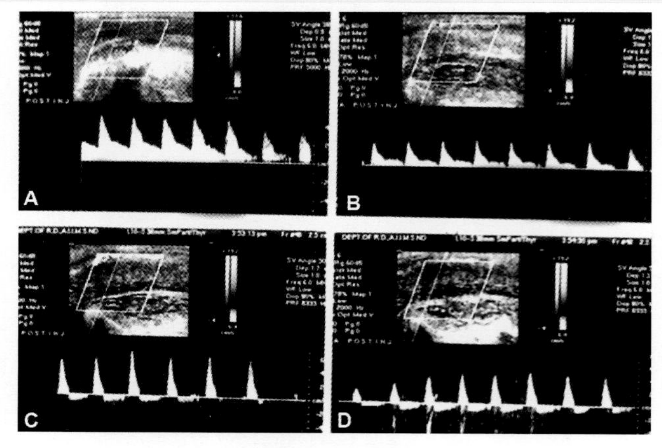

FIGURE 7.18

Serial spectral tracings during post-papaverine Doppler study shows various phases of flow pattern. Phase I (A): Increase in systolic and diastolic velocities; Phase II (B): Decrease in end-diastolic velocity with appearance of diachrotic notch; Phase III (C): Diastolic flow is reduced to zero or may be reversed; Phase IV: (D): Reduced peak systolic velocity with diastolic flow reversal

Note: Arterial erectile dysfunction, after prostaglandin injection will demonstrate a lower than normal peak systolic velocity during the tumescent phase. A PSV<25 cm/s in deep penile artery is definitely pathological. Values in the range of 25-35 cm/s borderline. The systolic upslope is markedly flattened resulting in a broadened, undulating spectral waveform.

Venous erectile dysfunction, detected indirectly by analyzing Doppler spectra recorded from deep penile arteries. Normal compression of draining venules by the increasing blood volume is manifested by decrease of forward diastolic flow or even reverse flow in deep penile artery. The resistance index value reaches higher than 1.0

Chapter Eight

Doppler in Small Parts and HRUS

RHABDOMYOSARCOMA

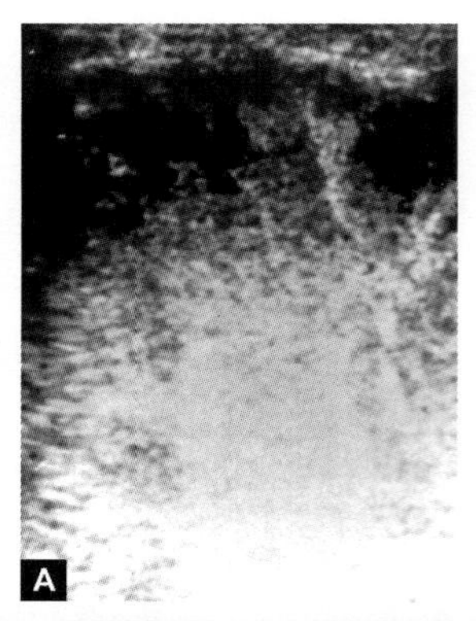

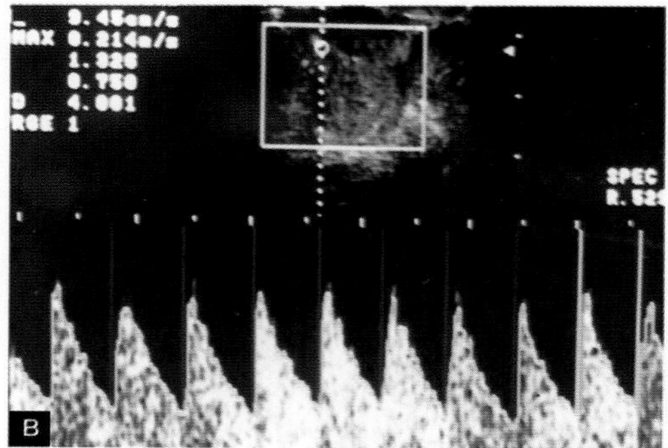

FIGURES 8.1A and B

(A) Gray scale image reveals a large heterogeneous mass in the neck in a child (B) Color and pulse Doppler image shows central, high velocity flow arterial flow with high pulsatility and high RI pattern in the lesion suggestive of a malignant lesion

SUBCUTANEOUS MASS IN RT ARM – METASTASIS

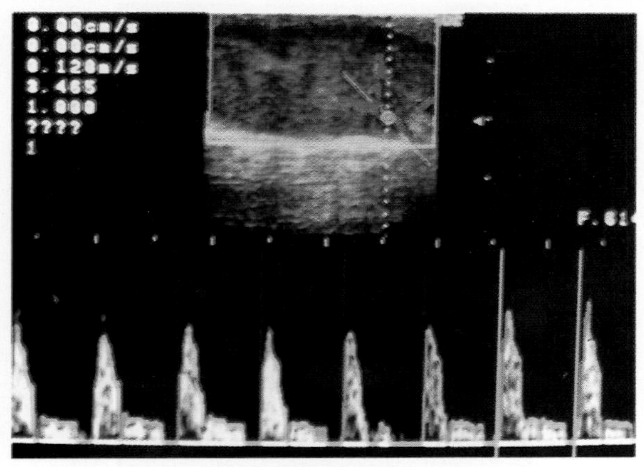

FIGURE 8.2

Color Doppler of right arm shows a subcutaneous mass with intralesional vascularity and central high velocity flow signal with high pulsatility and high RI pattern suggestive of a malignant lesion. The histological diagnosis was metastasis

BASAL CELL CARCINOMA

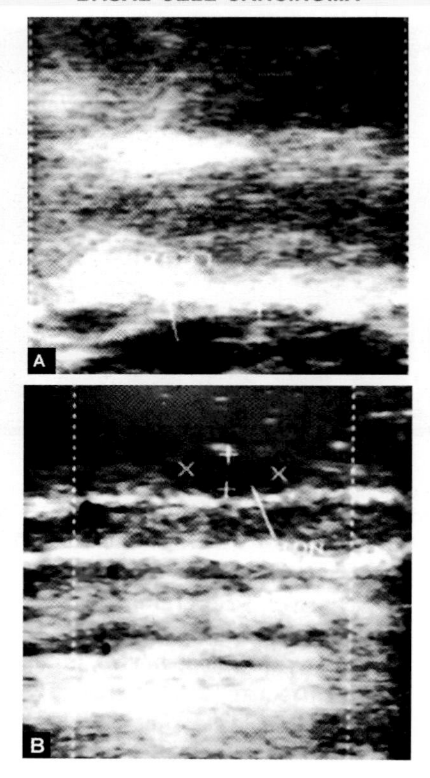

FIGURES 8.3A and B

A well-defined hypo to anechoic skin lesion seen on gray scale image. (A) Showing no vascularity on color Doppler image (B) Suggestive of absence of significant vascularity. This is useful prior to FNAC or biopsy as an OPD procedure

PYOGENIC GRANULOMA

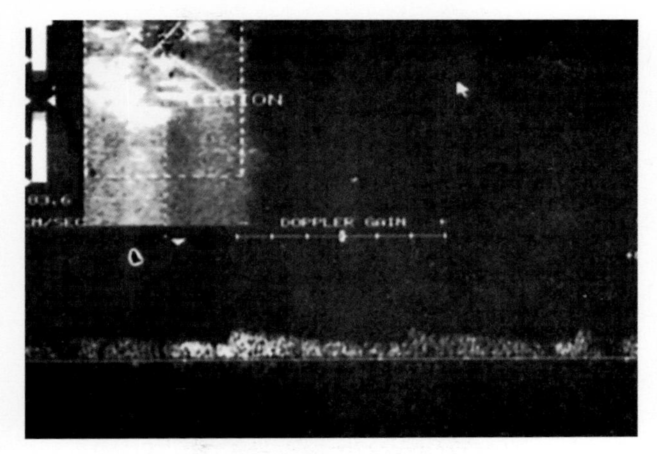

FIGURE 8.4

A well-defined hypoechoic skin lesion seen with Doppler analysis showing low systolic and end-diastolic velocity suggestive of a benign lesion

METASTASIS

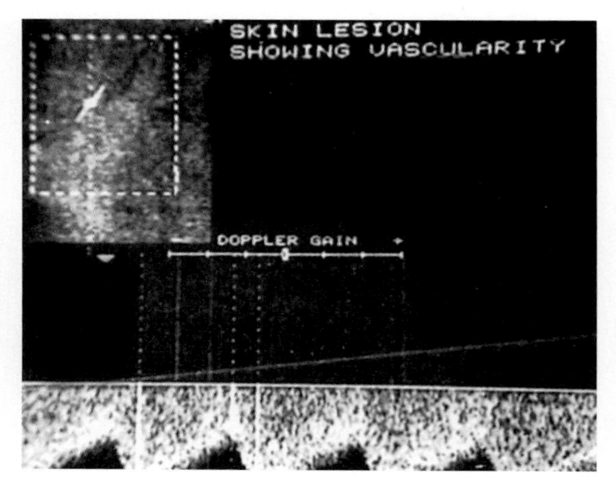

FIGURE 8.5

A large well-defined hypoechoic skin lesion is seen in the scalp from carcinoma thyroid showing a high systolic and end-diastolic velocity suggestive of a malignant lesion

SUPERFICIAL HEMANGIOMA (OF LIP)

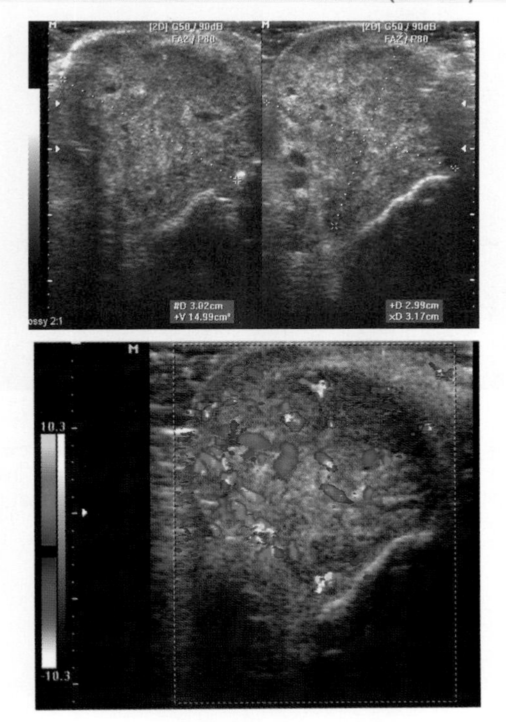

FIGURES 8.6A and B

(A) Gray scale image shows a mixed echogenic mass lesion with multiple tortuous channels suggestive of a possibility of vascular lesion, (B) Color Doppler shows numerous vessels within and at the periphery of lesion confirming hemangioma

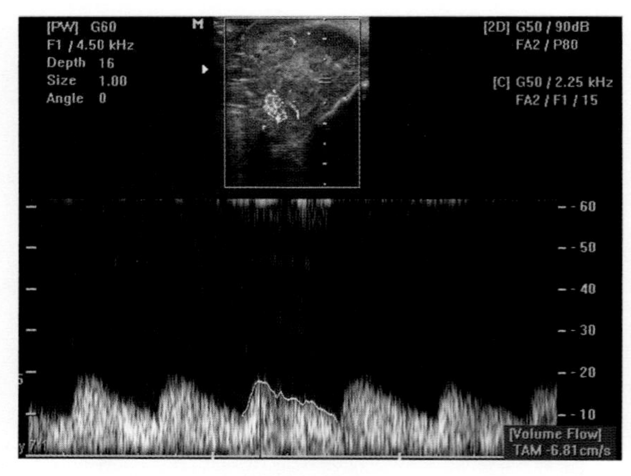

FIGURE 8.6C

Spectral flow shows low velocity and low resistance arterial flow within hemangioma s/o benign lesion. Such a vascular pattern also indicates that injury will lead to oozing rather than torrential bleeding that can be controlled by compression technique

ARTERIOVENOUS MALFORMATION IN THE LEG

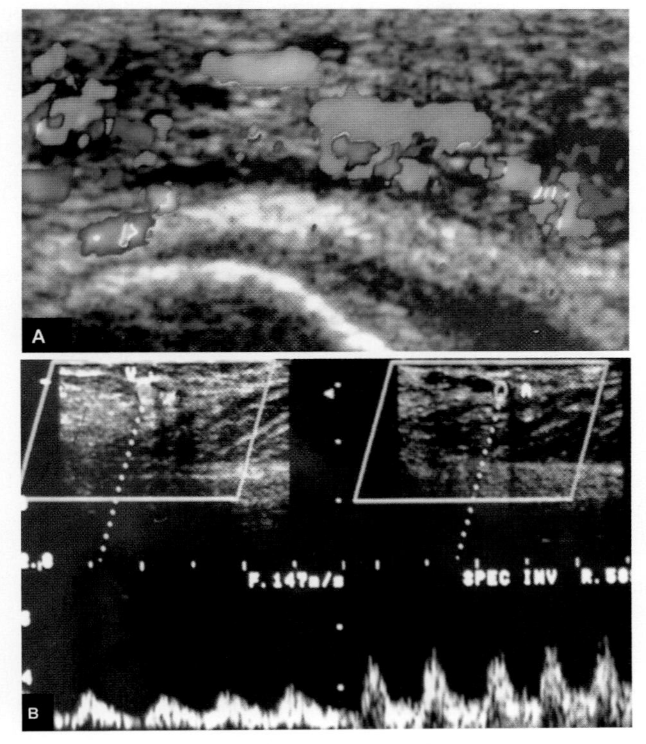

FIGURES 8.7A and B

(A) Color Doppler image shows multiple vascular spaces in a swelling of knee, (B) Spectral tracing shows arterialization of venous flow characteristic of AVM

CARCINOMA OF BREAST

These images show that carcinoma breast is not very vascular and may have variable pattern of vascularity due to intense desmoplastic reaction associated with it

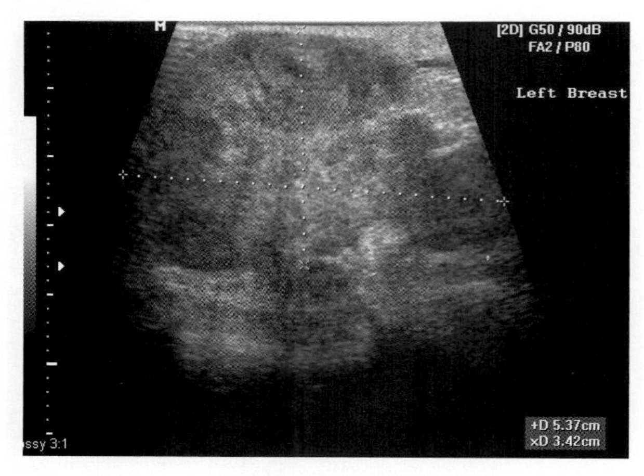

FIGURE 8.8A

Gray scale US shows a large irregular mass lesion in the breast

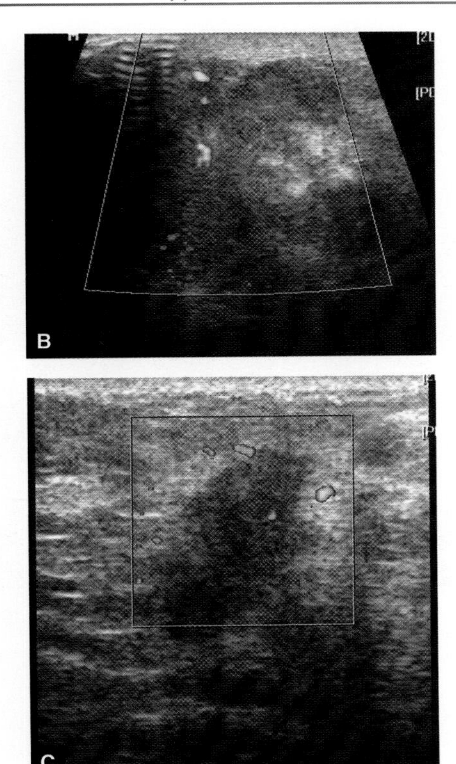

FIGURES 8.8B and C

(B) Power Doppler image shows blood vessels only at the periphery of lesion, (C) Color Doppler image in another case shows color signals located within the mass

THYROTOXICOSIS

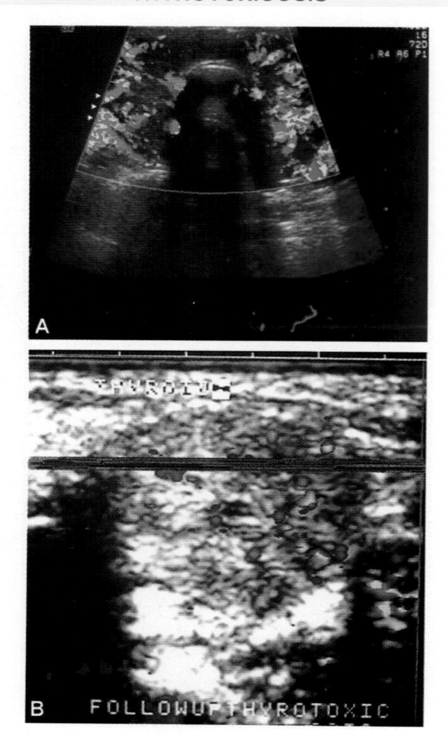

FIGURES 8.9A and B

(A) Color Doppler image in a case of thyrotoxicosis shows marked vascularity in both lobes of thyroid, the pattern known as the 'Thyroid inferno' sign, (B) Follow-up of the same patient while on therapy, shows marked decrease in intraparenchymal color flow within the thyroid gland, suggesting good response to therapy

FOLLICULAR ADENOMA OF THYROID

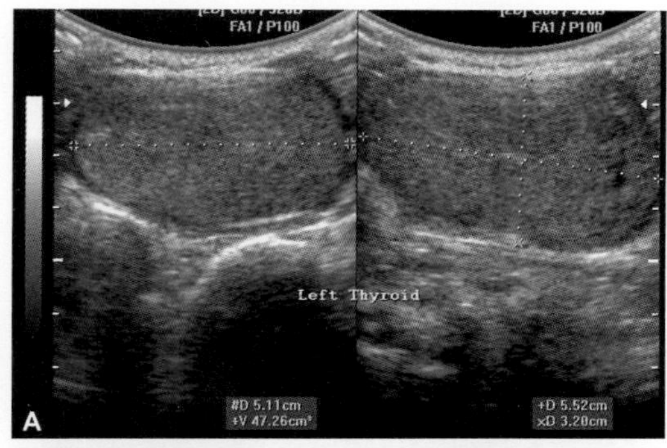

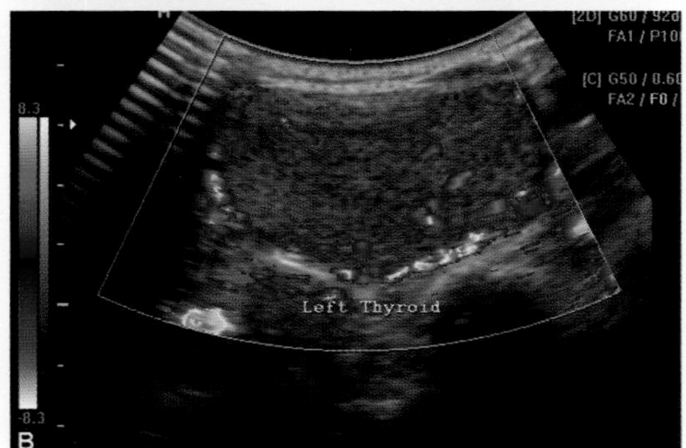

FIGURES 8.10A and B

(A) Gray scale image shows a well defined, solitary nodule in thyroid. Hypoechoic halo is visible around the nodule characteristic of benign lesion, (B) Doppler image reveals color flow corresponding to the halo with mild internal vascularity, thus confirming the diagnosis

FUNCTIONING NODULE - THYROID

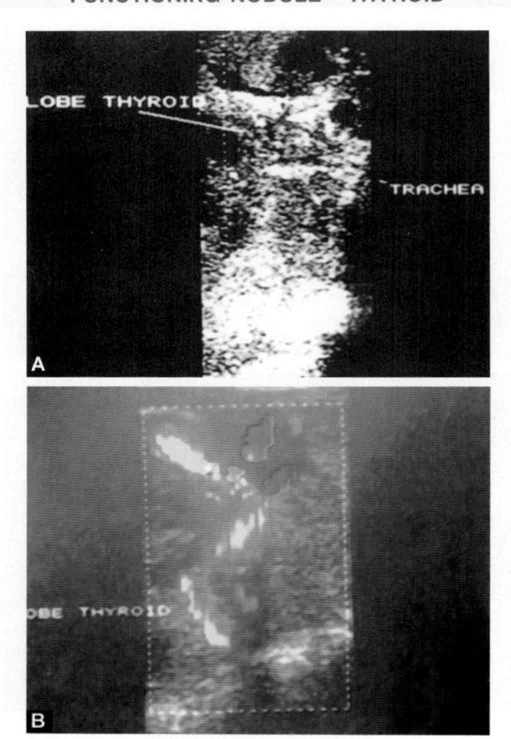

FIGURES 8.11A and B

(A) Gray scale image shows heterogeneous parenchyma of thyroid gland with obscuration of the anatomical planes, (B) Color Doppler image in a thyroid nodule shows evidence of both peripheral and central hypervascularity consistent with functioning nodule

PARATHYROID ADENOMA

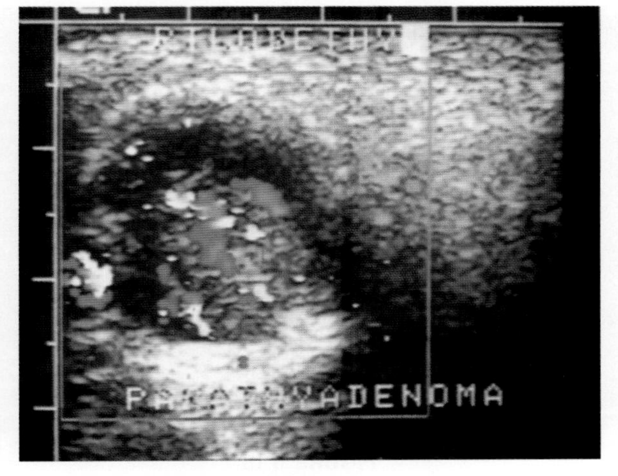

FIGURE 8.12

Color Doppler image of neck in a patient with clinical and biochemical evidence of hyperparathyroidism. A rounded mass lesion is seen posterior to the thyroid gland with increased vascularity seen on CDFI. On surgery, an adenoma was resected

BENIGN PAROTID MASS

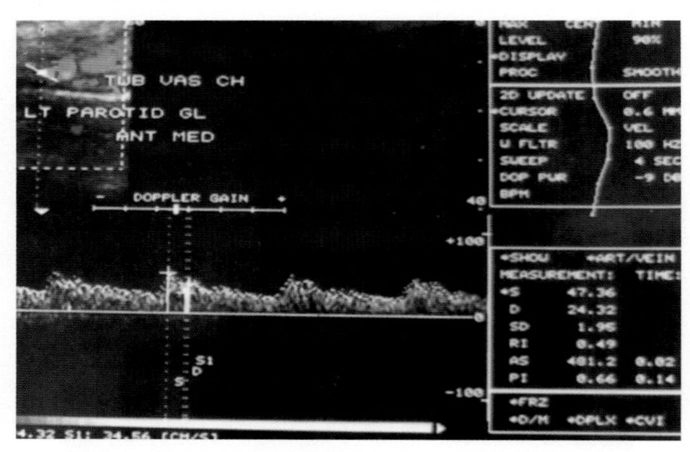

FIGURE 8.13

Color Doppler image in a benign parotid lesion shows a mass lesion with vascular channels. Few vascular channels show continuous venous flow, arterial waveform shows peak velocity 47.36 and mean RI 0.49 s/o benign lesion. Presence of RI < 0.8 and PI < 1.8 virtually excludes malignancy

PAROTID HEMANGIOMA

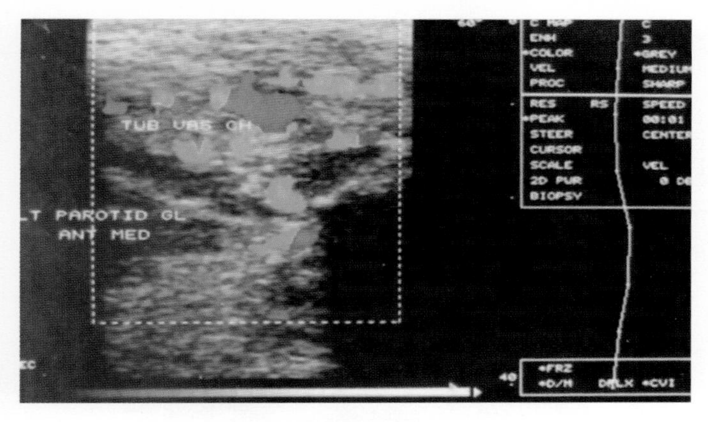

FIGURE 8.14

Color Doppler image shows a mass lesion with multiple vascular color flow signals

OCULAR MELANOMA

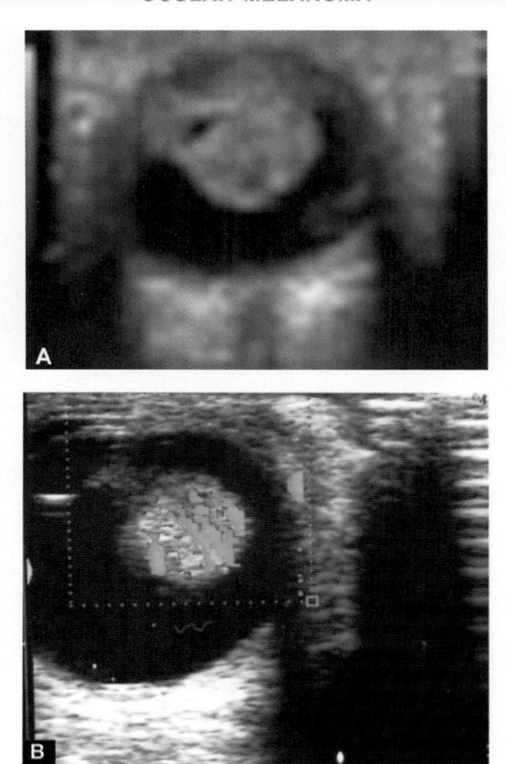

FIGURES 8.15A and B

(A) Gray scale image shows choroidal mass with fine calcification, (B) Color Doppler image reveals high vascularity within the mass. Melanoma was confirmed at histopathologic examination

RETINOBLASTOMA

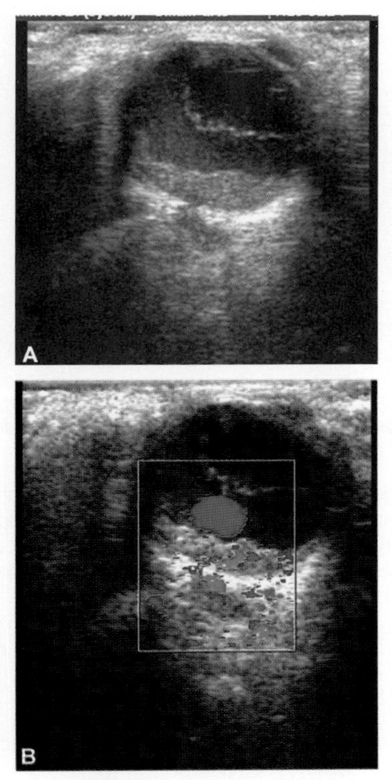

FIGURES 8.16A and B

(A) Gray scale image of the globe in a child shows a mass lesion in the region of retina. Calcification is also seen within the lesion along with retinal detachment, (B) CDFI shows a hyper-vascular lesion, suggesting malignant nature. On surgery, retinoblastoma was found

INTRAOCULAR HEMANGIOMA

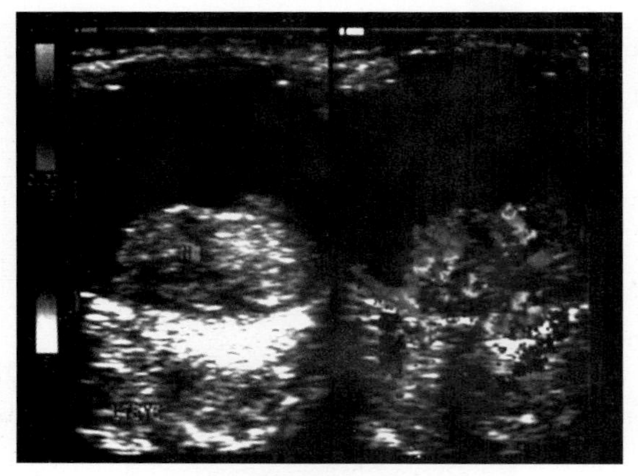

FIGURE 8.17

Gray scale image on left side shows a well-defined echogenic mass in the posterior part of the globe with posterior acoustic enhancement. Color Doppler image on the right side shows high vascularity within the lesion suggestive of hemangioma (proved on histopathology of surgically removed tumor)

LIPOMA

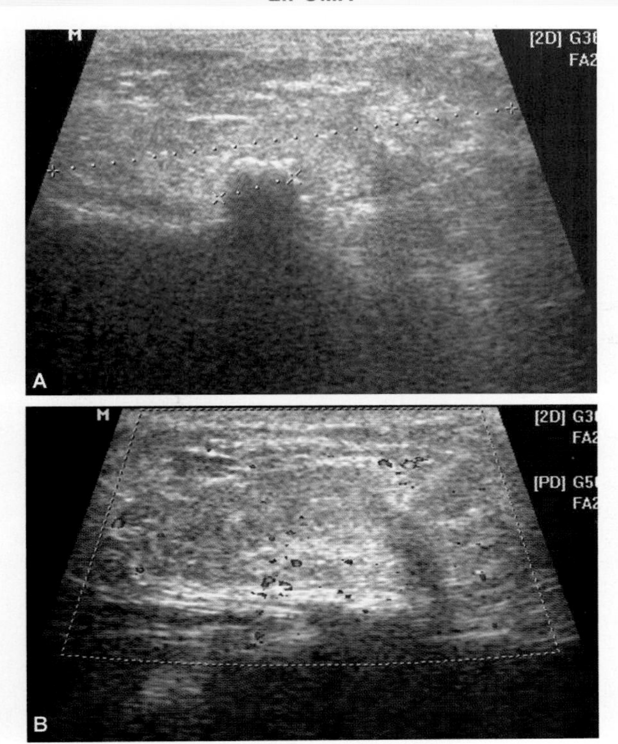

FIGURES 8.18A and B

(A) Gray scale image shows a solid echogenic lesion with a focus of calcification in the subcutaneous tissues with no obvious vascularity on power Doppler imaging, (B) Suggestive of lipoma (proved on CT by presence of fat attenuation)

CAPILLARY HEMANGIOMA

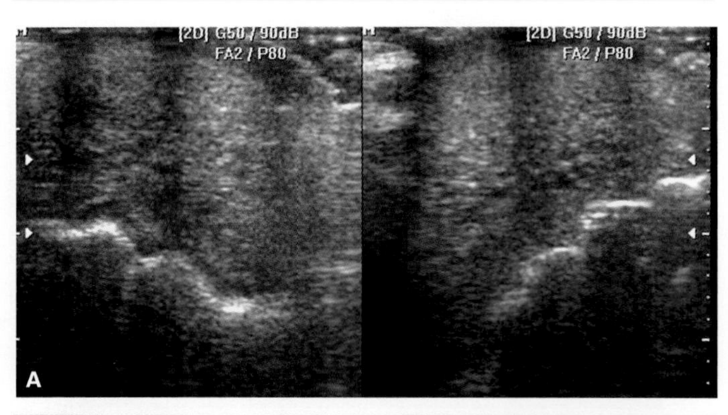

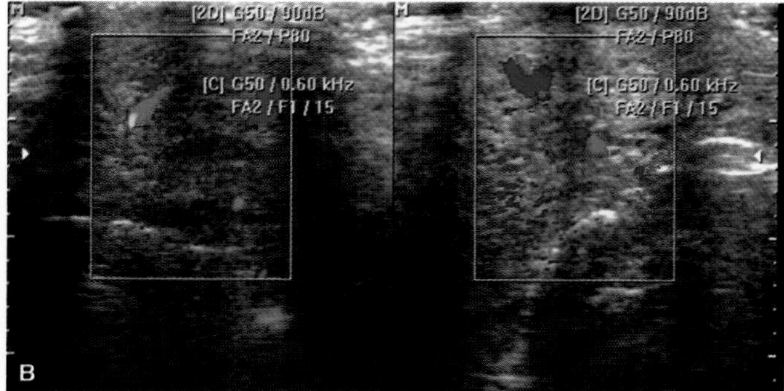

FIGURES 8.19A and B

(A) Gray scale image shows an enlarged tongue with numerous minute spaces (B) Some of them showing blood flow on CDFI

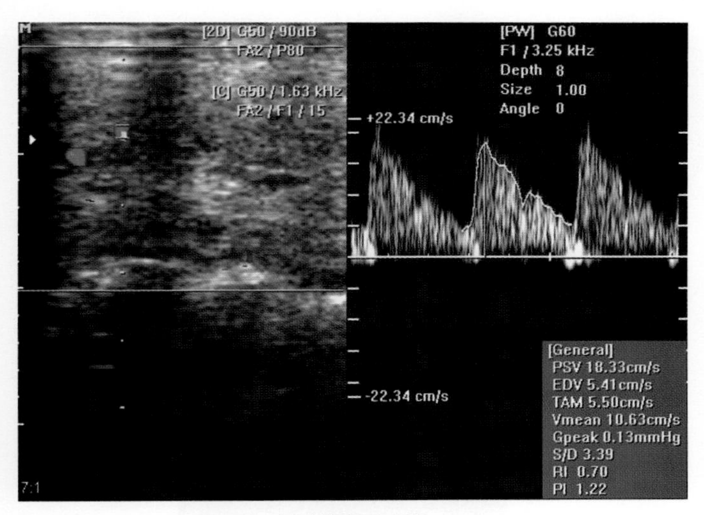

FIGURE 8.19C

Presence of arterial flow with moderate RI and PI on spectral Doppler

FIBROADENOMA

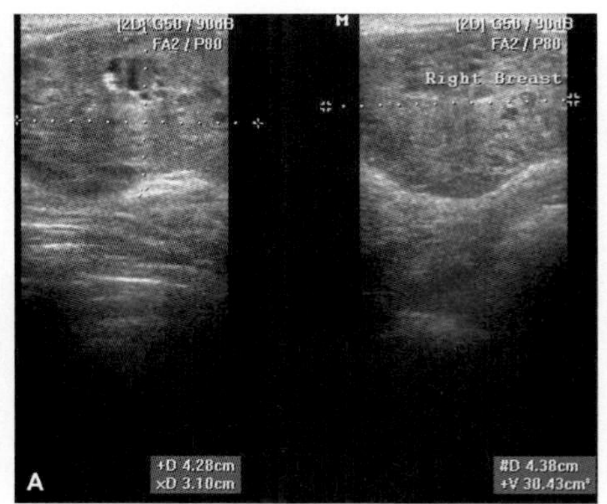

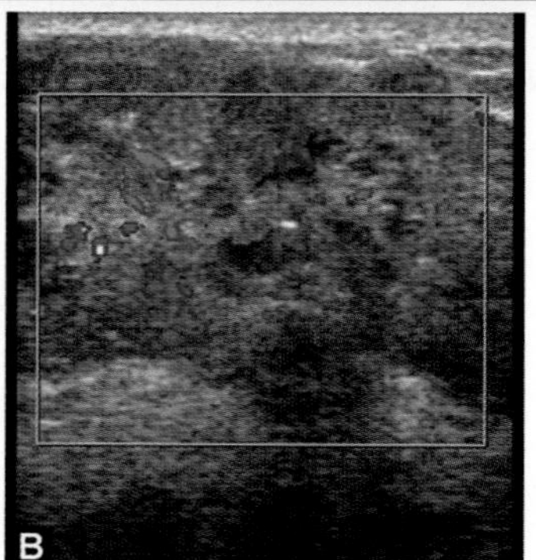

FIGURES 8.20A and B

(A) Gray scale image shows a large fibroadenoma with cystic degeneration and calcification with high central vascularity on CDFI (B) This pattern is seen in fibroadenoma when it is undergoing degeneration or necrosis

INFILTRATING CARCINOMA

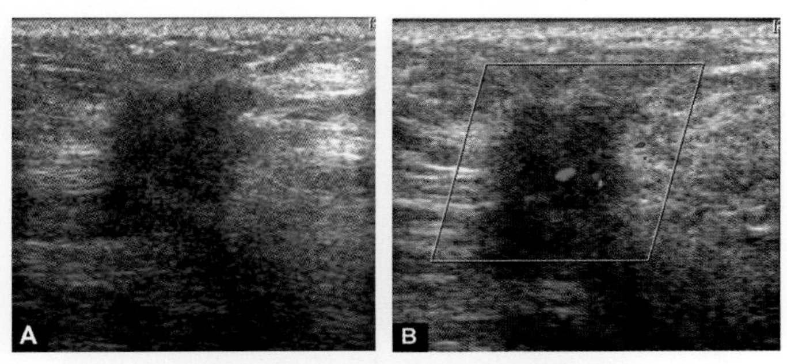

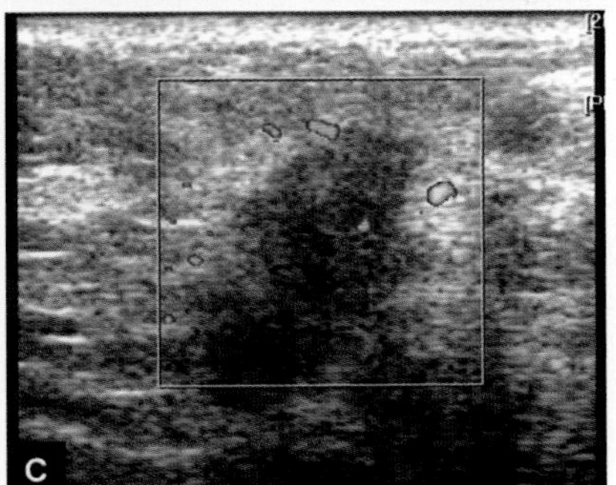

FIGURES 8.21A to C

(A) Gray scale image shows an infiltrating carcinoma with very low central and peripheral vascularity on both CDFI, (B) And PDI, (C) Suggestive of relatively avascular nature of these lesions

SUBMANDIBULAR GLAND ABSCESS

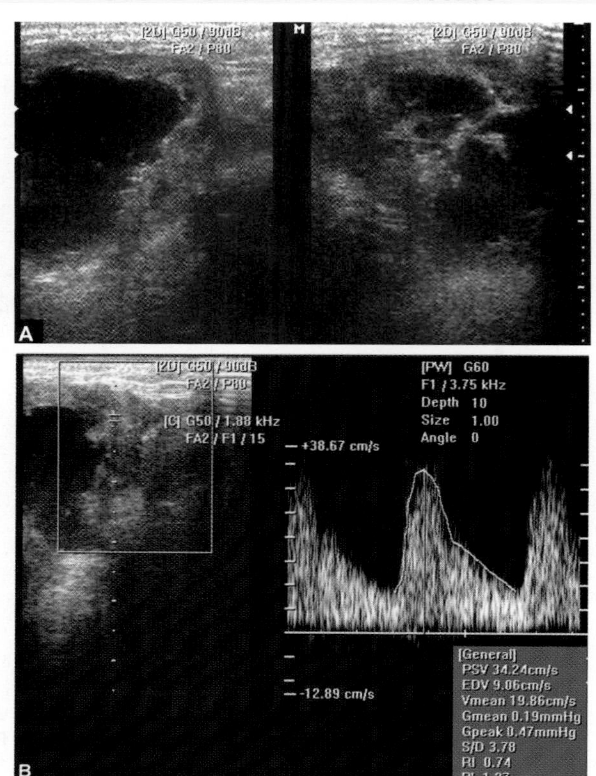

FIGURES 8.22A and B

(A) Gray scale image shows a complex mass with thickened wall. (B) Mild peripheral vascularity with moderate RI and PSV is noted in CDFI (Proven case)

GRANULOMATOUS PAROTITIS (PROVEN CASE)

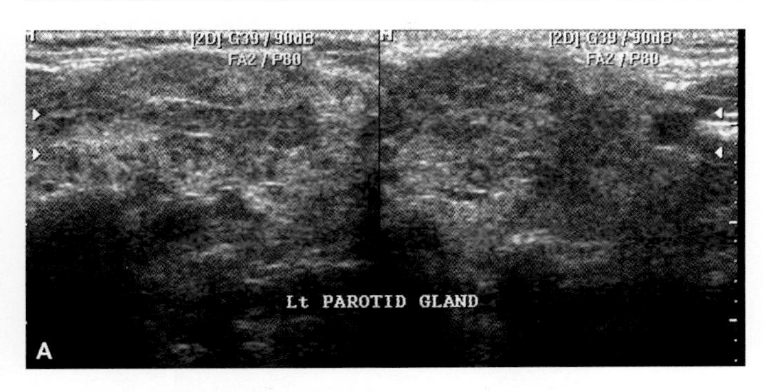

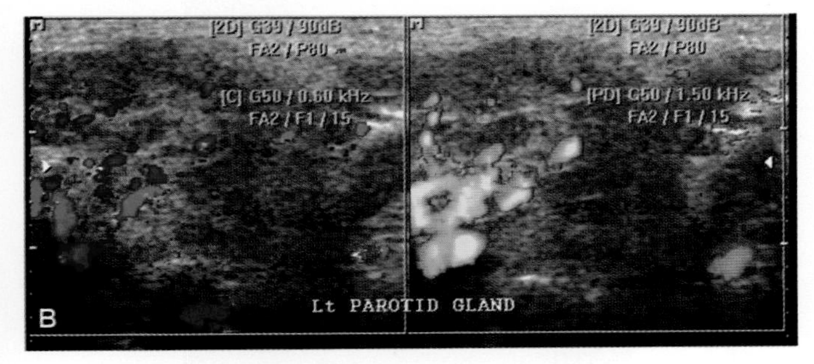

FIGURES 8.23A and B

(A) Gray scale image shows heterogeneous echotexture of parotid gland with, (B) High vascularity on both CDFI and PDI without any discrete lesion

ACUTE APPENDICITIS

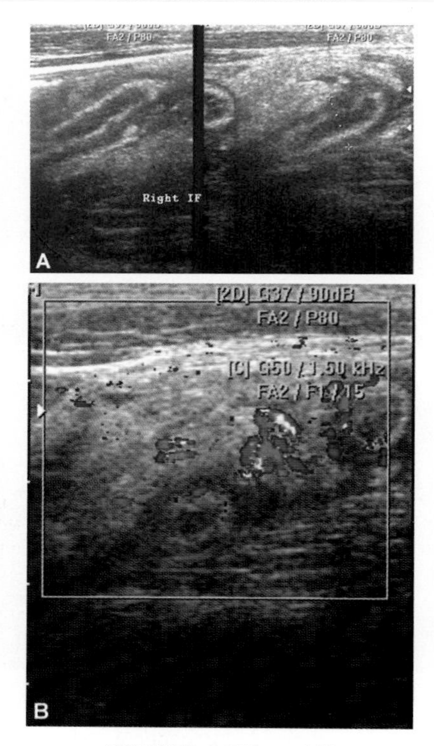

FIGURES 8.24A and B

(A) Gray scale image shows dilated appendix with thickened walls and echogenic mucosa and surrounding echogenic edematous mesentery (B) Color Doppler image shows high vascularity in the region of appendix and mesentery suggestive of inflammation. The lesions were surgically proved to be a case of acute appendicitis

GASTRIC ADENOCARCINOMA

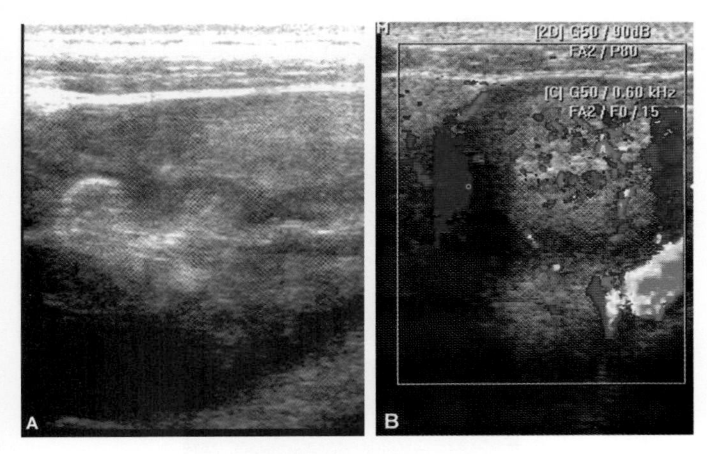

FIGURES 8.25A and B

(A) Gray scale image shows thickened gastric wall in the region of antrum, (B) Color Doppler image shows very high vascularity with haphazard arrangement of vessels suggestive of malignant etiology

RECTAL ADENOCARCINOMA

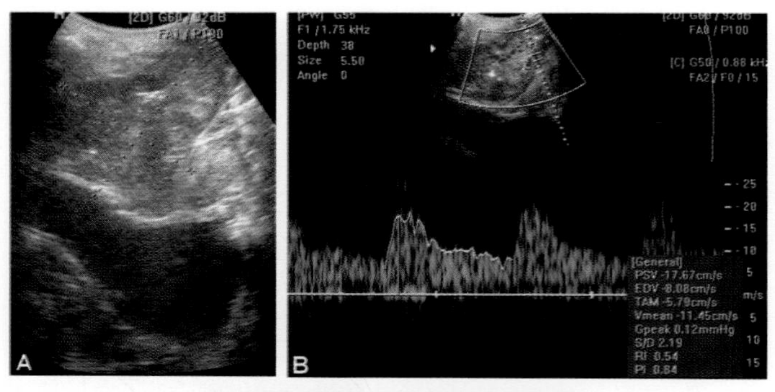

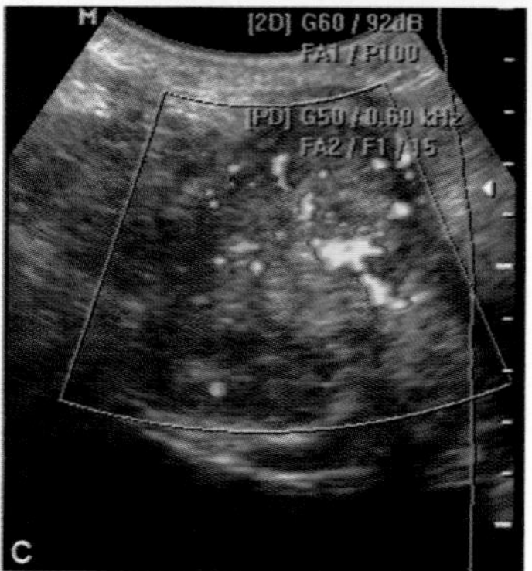

FIGURES 8.26A to C

(A) Gray scale image shows lobulated mass posterior to bladder on transperineal US, (B) Color Doppler image shows very high internal and peripheral vascularity with low RI and PI values suggestive of malignant etiology, (C) Power Doppler image shows pattern similar to CDFI

ADENITIS – INFLAMMATORY

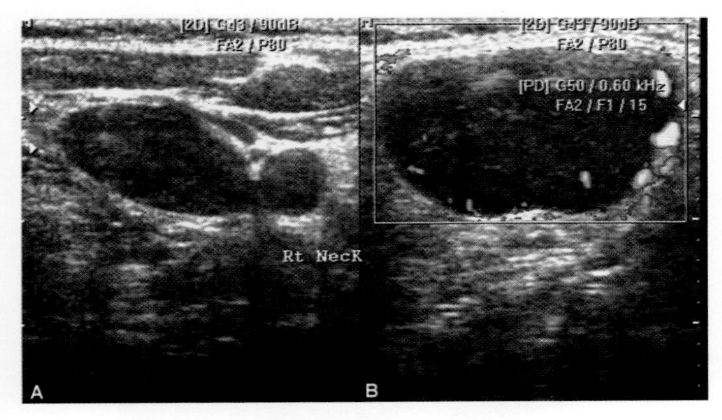

FIGURES 8.27A and B

Gray scale image (A) and power Doppler image (B) shows enlarged necrotic node with posterior acoustic enhancement with mild peripheral vascularity suggestive of inflammatory (probably tubercular) adenitis (FNAC proved)

PROSTATITIS

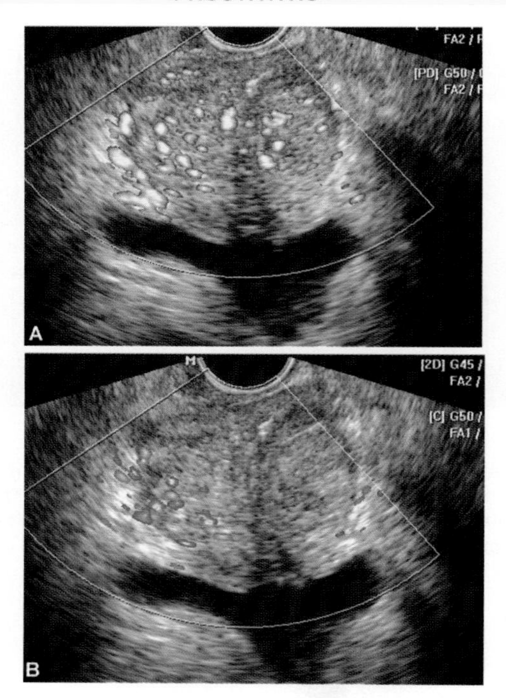

FIGURES 8.28A and B

Normal pattern of power Doppler (A) and color Doppler (B) flow of prostate as seen on TRUS with mild intraparenchymal and peripheral vascularity. Peripheral vascularity corresponds to prostatic venous plexus

GRAVES DISEASE IN 28 YEARS MALE

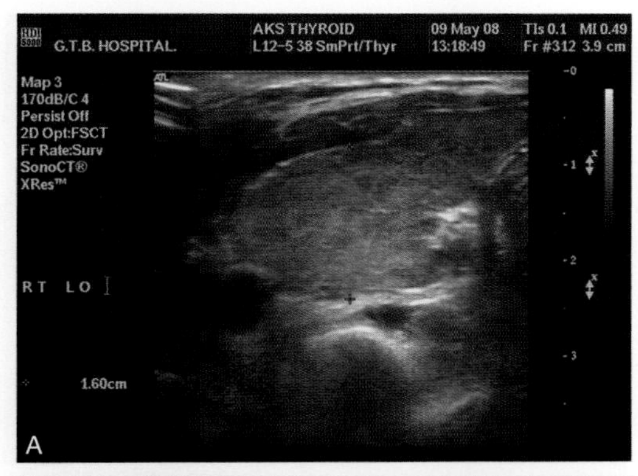

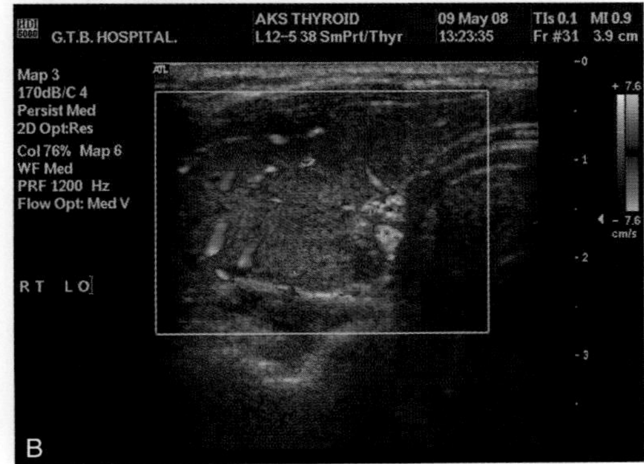

FIGURES 8.29A and B

(A) Right lobe of thyroid gland showing multiple hypoechoic areas. (B) Right lobe of thyroid showing increased vascularity. This was diagnosed as graves disease on anti thyroid antibody examination

ANAPLASTIC CARCINOMA IN 80 YEARS FEMALE

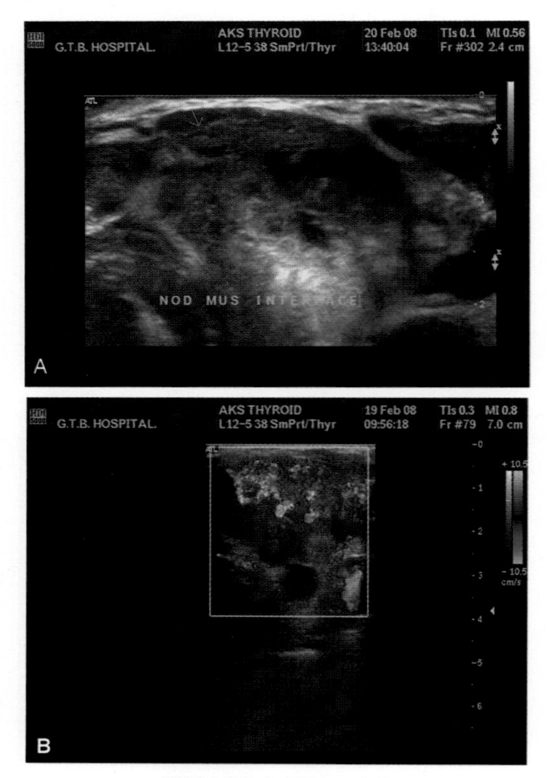

FIGURES 8.30A and B

(A) A large nodule in left lobe of thyroid infiltrating in strap muscles. (B) The nodule is showing markedly increased intranodular vascularity

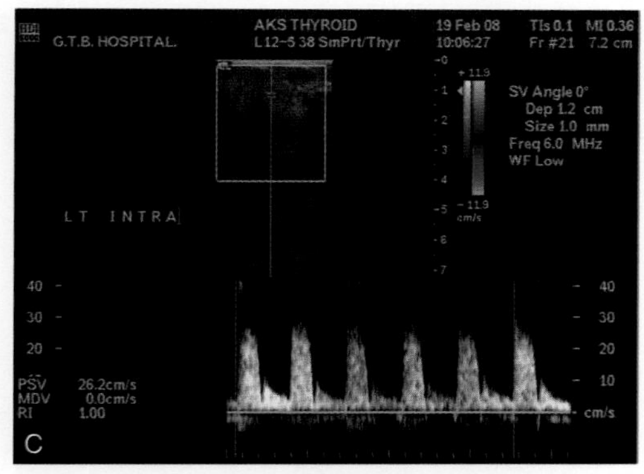

FIGURE 8.30C

The nodule has low resistance flow suggestive of malignant change. This came out to be anaplastic carcinoma on histopathological examination

METASTATIC LYMPH NODES IN 60 YEARS FEMALE

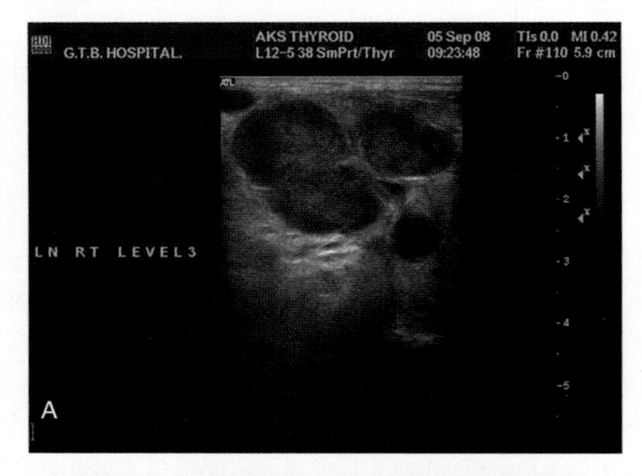

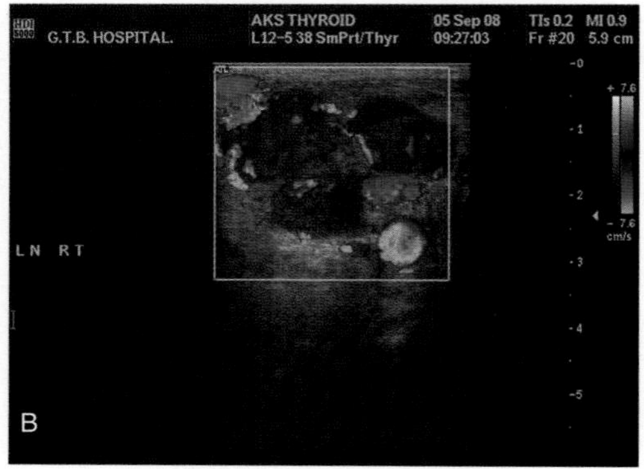

FIGURES 8.31A and B

(A) Multiple welldefined round hypoechoic level 2 lymph nodes. (B) The lymph nodes showing increased vascularity. These were metastatic lymph nodes from papillary carcinoma thyroid

Note:

Lymph Node Evaluation:

- During B-Mode, the size, shape (M/T Ratio), margins, central hila echo, and echogenicity have to be seen.
- During Color Duplex evaluation, see the degree of vascularity, vascular distribution pattern, and pulsatility of intranodal blood flow.

Normal lymph nodes have characteristic features as:

1. Size < 1.5 cm
2. Sharp margin
3. Oblong shape (M/T ratio > 2)
4. Bright hilar echo
5. No detectable vascularity in color – flow image

Malignant lymphoma has the following features:

1. Spherical shape (M/T RATIO < 2)
2. Sharp margins
3. Frequent absence of Hilar echo
4. Marked low echogenicity
5. Marked Hypervasculrity
6. Arborizing intranodal vascular pattern
7. Intranodal RI < 0.8.

Lymph nodes metastasis from squamous cell carcinoma (SCC) has got characteristic features as – spherical shape (M/T ratio < 2), ill-defined margins with hypoechoic, regressive change, no Hilar echo; vascular pattern is irregular with intranodal RI > 0.8, scant vascularity—moderately vascularized in relation to size, the vessel radiating from periphery of the node towards centre. This spoke wheel pattern of vascularity is always pathological.

Lymphadenitis

Acute	*Chronic*
1. Oblong shape (M/T ratio >> 2)	Oblong shape (M/T ratio >> 2)
2. Cortex slightly hypo-echoic	Cortex slightly hypoechoic
3. Central hilar echo	Central hilar echo
4. Sharp margins	Sharp margins
5. Hypervascularity	No detectable vascularity
6. Central hilar vessel	-----------
7. Intra-nodal RI < 0.8	-----------

Note: The great vascularity of acute lymphadenitis is the only feature that distinguishes it from chronic lymphadenitis. A lymph node in chronic lymphadenitis differs from a normal lymph node only in its size.

CHAPTER NINE

Doppler in Peripheral Arteries

NORMAL PERIPHERAL ARTERY WAVEFORM

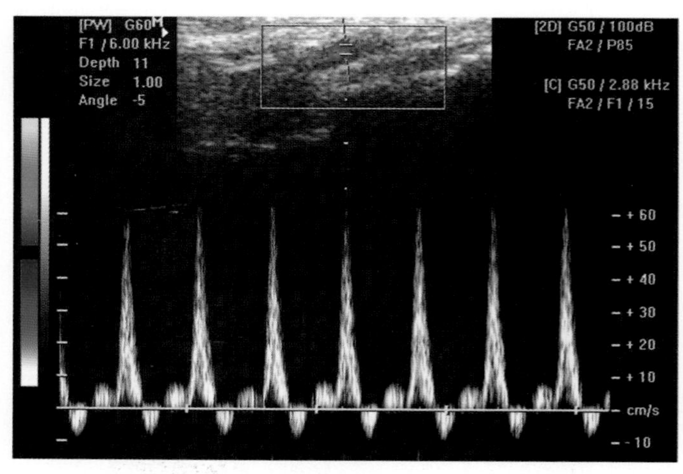

FIGURE 9.1

Duplex Doppler tracing from peripheral artery showing a typical triphasic waveform with forward systolic, reverse diastolic and forward diastolic flow suggestive of high pulsatility and high resistance flow

THROMBOSIS OF SUPERFICIAL FEMORAL ARTERY

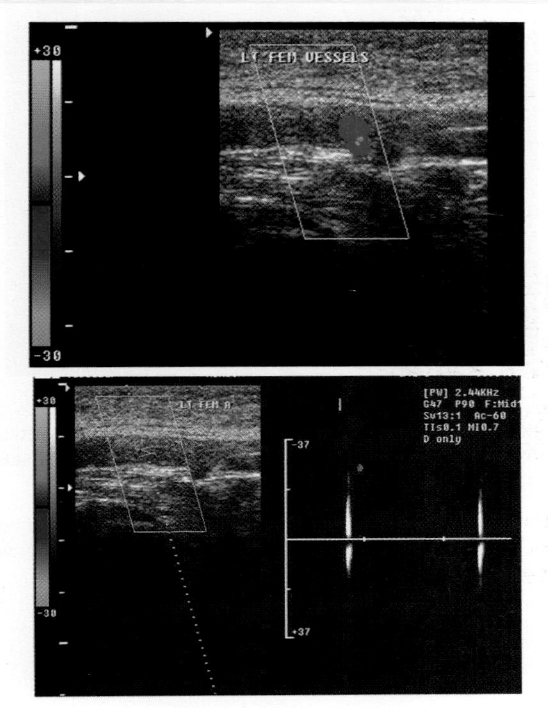

FIGURES 9.2A and B

(A) Color Doppler image shows minimal color flow with echogenic material filling the lumen of artery suggestive of subacute thrombus obstructing the flow of the artery (B) Pulse Doppler shows markedly attenuated waveform with near complete absence of flow

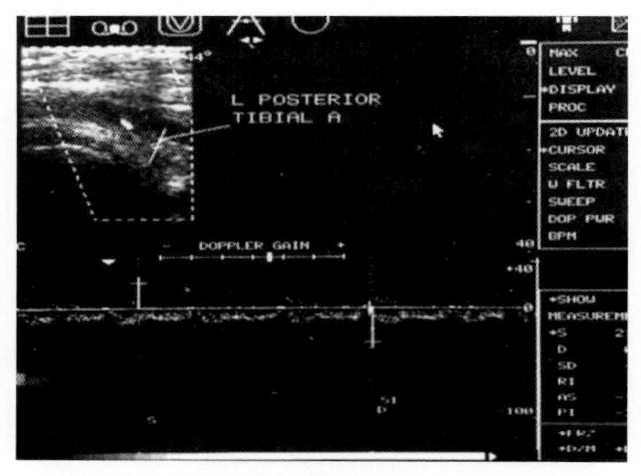

FIGURE 9.2C

Spectral tracing from posterior tibial artery shows rising delayed systolic peak with low amplitude and low velocity continuous end-diastolic flow characteristic of tardus—parvus waveform

ACUTE THROMBUS

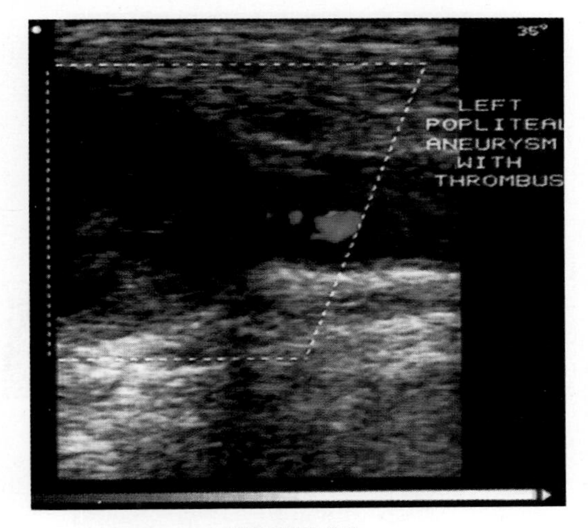

FIGURE 9.3

Color Doppler flow image at the level of popliteal artery shows fusiform dilatation on the left side of the image suggesting presence of an aneurysm with no demonstrable color flow suggestive of acute thrombosis. Acute thrombus appears anechoic

PSEUDOANEURYSM OF ARTERY

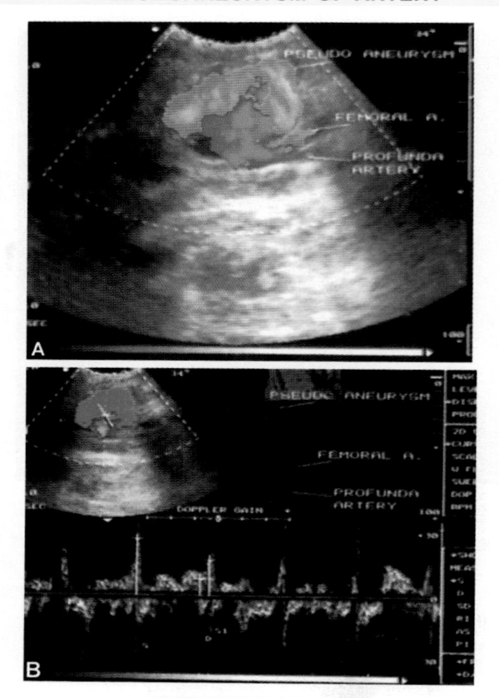

FIGURES 9.4A and B

(A) Color Doppler image shows a cystic mass with swirling colors, i.e. presence of multiple colors simultaneously instead of the arterial or venous color pattern known as 'ying-yang sign' characteristic of pseudoaneurysm of an artery, (B) Spectral Doppler shows bi-directional, haphazard blood flow that neither conforms to arterial nor venous pattern, known as 'to and fro' sign

ARTERIOVENOUS FISTULA

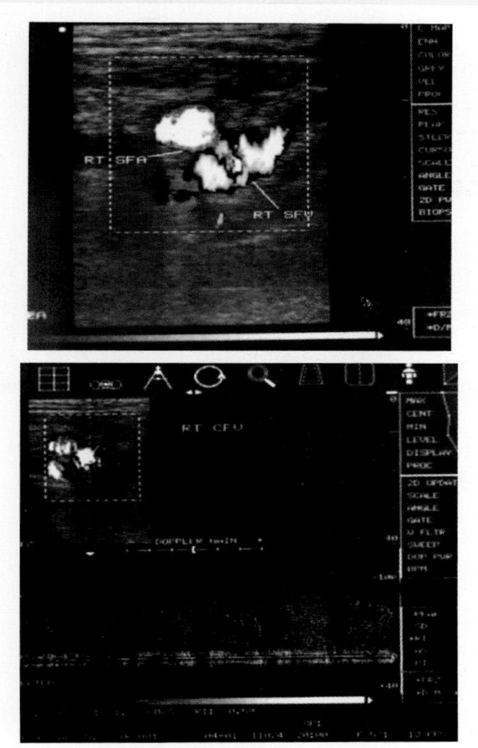

FIGURES 9.5A and B

(A) Color Doppler image at the level of upper thigh shows a communication between superficial femoral artery and vein with varying colors, (B) Pulse Doppler in common femoral vein shows turbulent high velocity waveform that is characteristic of arterialization of venous flow

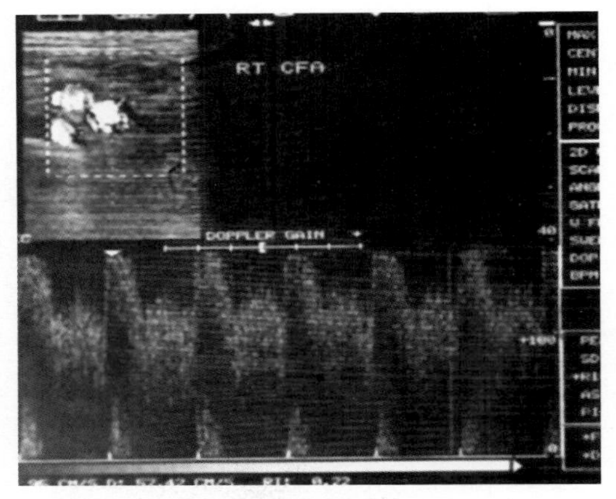

FIGURE 9.5C

Pulse Doppler in common femoral artery shows persistent antegrade flow in diastole that is characteristic of venous flow

ARTERIOSCLEROSIS

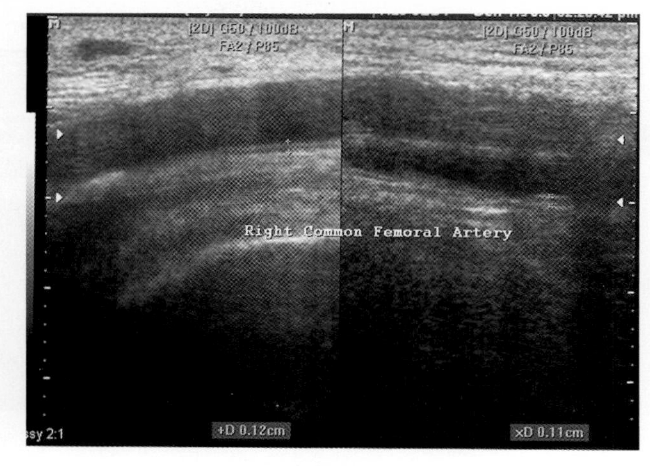

FIGURE 9.6

Gray scale image showing thickening of the intima media complex in the common femoral artery with echogenic intimal surface suggestive of arteriosclerosis as seen in hypertension, diabetes and vasculitis

RECANALIZATION OF CHRONIC THROMBUS IN ARTERY

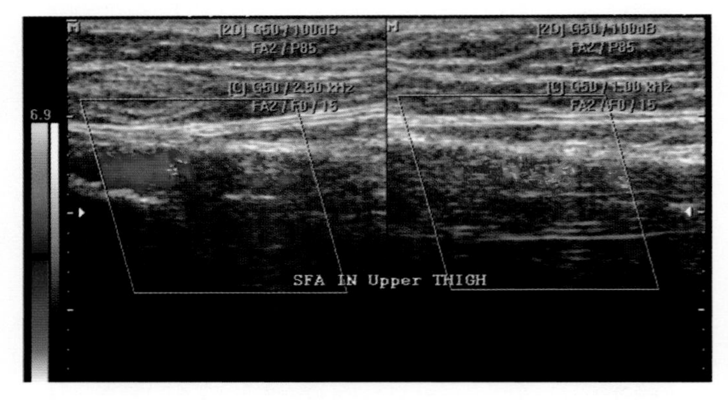

FIGURE 9.7

Color Doppler image shows fragmented color flow pattern in the superficial femoral artery along with echogenic material in the lumen suggestive of partial recanalization of chronic thrombus in the artery

Spectral analysis criteria for different % stenosis

Percent stenosis	*Prestenotic spectrum*	*Intrastenotic spectrum*	*Spectrum just past the stenosis*	*Spectrum far distal to the stenosis*
0-50%	Normal: -Triphasic or biphasic -Narrow frequency band -Clear spectral window	-Increase in PSV (by <100% and/or <180 cm/s)	-No significant turbulence -Possible flow reversal	-Same as prestenotic
51-75%	Normal	-Increase in PSV (>100% and/or >180 cm/s) -Slight decrease in pulsatility	-Flow reversal -Possible slight turbulence -Some fill-in of spectral window	-Pulsatility normal or slightly reduced
76-99%	-Normal or slightly reduced velocity -Pulsatility increased	-Increase in PSV (<250% and/or >180 cm/s) -Pulsatility decreased	-Significant turbulence -Complete fill-in of spectral window	-Reduced PSV -Reduced pulsatility -Flattened systolic peak
100%	-Low velocity -Increased pulsatility -Narrow complex with high reverse flow component	-No flow signal	Slight flow in distal connecting vessel due to collaterals	-Very flat systolic peak

ABI = ankle pressure/systolic arm pressure
AAPG = systolic arm pressure - ankle pressure

ABI	*AAPG*	*Interpretation*
>12	< -20 mm Hg	Suspicion of Monckeberg sclerosis (reducing the compressibility of the vessels)
>0.97	between 0 and -20 mm Hg	Normal
0.7-0.97	between + 5 and + 20 mm Hg	Vascular stenosis or well-collateralized occlusions, suspicion of PAOD
< 0.69	>20 mm Hg	Suspicion of poorly collateralized occlusions and multilevel occlusions

Note:

Overestimation or underestimation measurements are the usual error in Doppler pressure measurements. Overestimation or over pressure may be due to hypertension, ankle edema, chronic venous insufficiency, positioning the upper body too high, and Monckeberg sclerosis.

Underestimation of pressure may be due to excessive probe pressure, insufficient rest period, deflating the cuff too rapidly, stenosis between the cuff and probe and hypertension of the ankle joint

Criteria for bypass stenosis
PSV < 45 cm/s
PSV > 250 cm/s
Change in the PSV ratio of > 2,5 (most reliable parameter for stenoses > 50% (7.7)

Recurrent stenosis are due to
a. Acutre thrombosis
b. Infection
c. Myointimal hyperplasia
d. Vascular dissection after PTA due to intimal-medial tears
e. Improperly dilated stent
f. Irregularities at the junction of the bypass or stent with the blood vessel

Formula for calculating flow in a hemodialysis fistula		
Vol=	$\pi \cdot r^2 \cdot V_{mean} \cdot 60$	
Vol=	Volume flow in ml/min	
r	=	Radius (1/2 diameter) in cm
V_{mean}	=	Average flow velocity in cm/s (V_{mean} represents the time averaged velocity, not the average peak velocity)

CHAPTER TEN

Doppler in Peripheral Veins

NORMAL PERIPHERAL VENOUS WAVEFORM

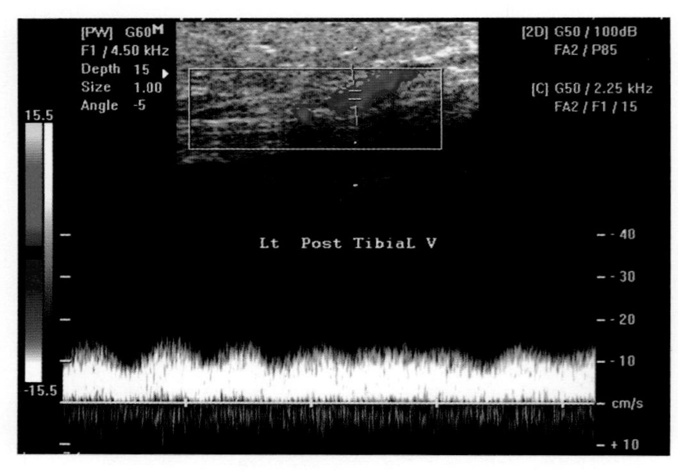

FIGURE 10.1

Color Doppler image shows low velocity monophasic flow with respiratory variation (phasicity)

DEMONSTRATION OF COMPRESSIBILITY OF NORMAL VEIN

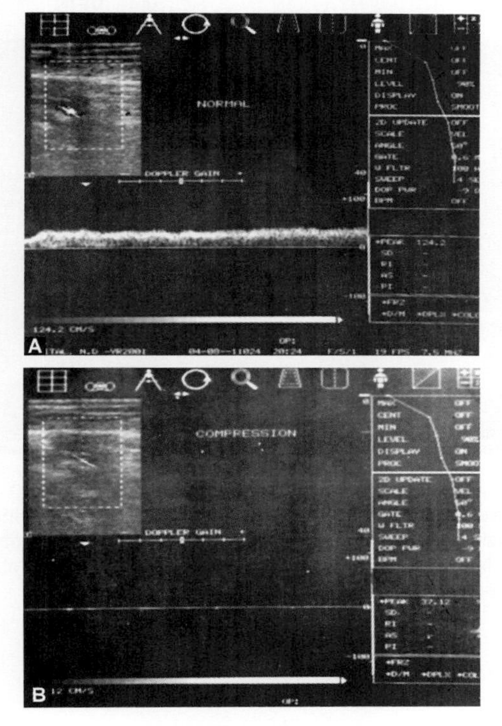

FIGURES 10.2A and B

(A) Duplex Doppler image shows common femoral vein (arrowhead) with low velocity monophasic flow, (B) On applying gentle transducer pressure, venous lumen is obliterated and there is complete cessation of flow

DEMONSTRATION OF DISTAL AUGMENTATION IN A NORMAL VEIN

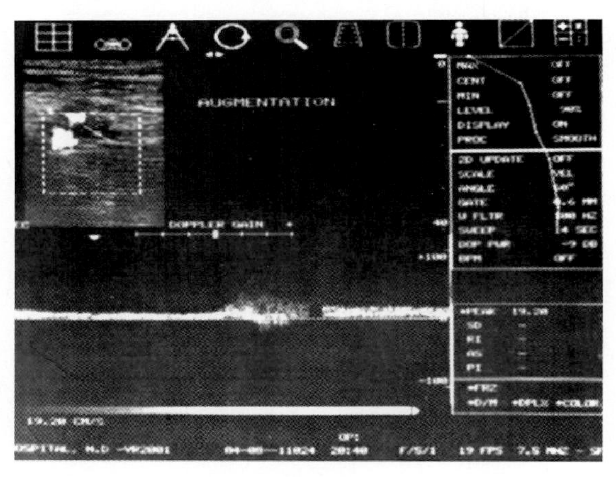

FIGURE 10.3

Longitudinal duplex Doppler image of femoral vein showing normal monophasic flow on the left side of trace with increased flow or augmentation of blood flow (arrow) on compression of distal lower limb seen on the right side of the Doppler trace

DEMONSTRATION OF EFFECT OF VALSALVA MANEUVER ON NORMAL VEIN

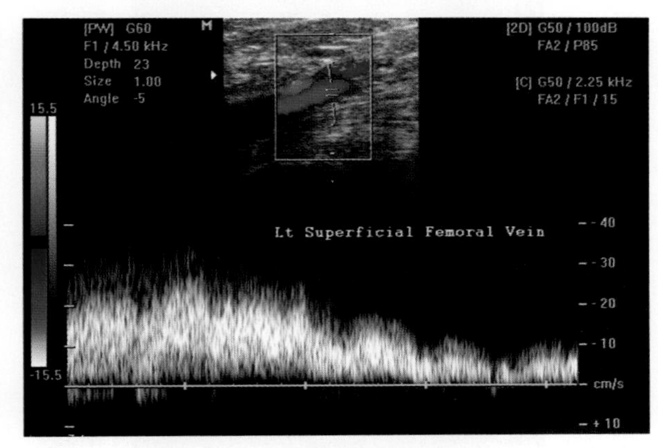

FIGURE 10.4

Longitudinal pulse Doppler image of superficial femoral vein showing progressive decrease in venous flow on performing Valsalva maneuver as seen on the right side of the trace

ACUTE THROMBUS IN VEIN

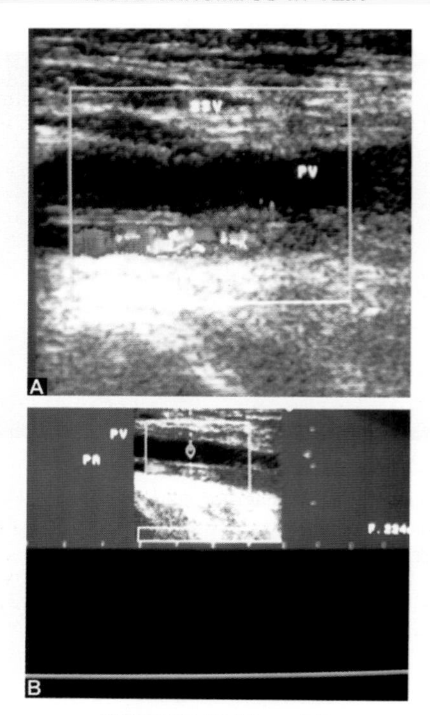

FIGURES 10.5A and B

(A) Color Doppler image in a patient with limb swelling shows enlarged popliteal vein with complete absence of color indicating acute thrombus. Acute thrombus is anechoic and there will be associated loss of the compressibility of vein and loss of respiratory passivity in distal veins (B) Spectral tracing from the vein revealed complete absence of flow indicating complete obstruction by an acute thrombus

DEEP VENOUS THROMBOSIS

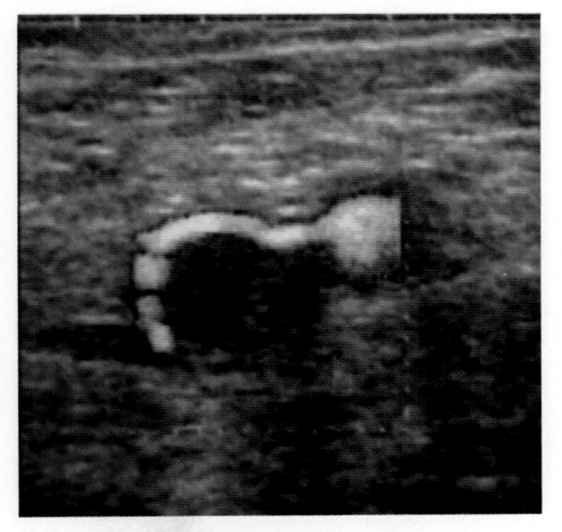

FIGURE 10.6

Power Doppler image in a case of deep vein thrombosis shows partial canalization of lumen at the periphery of the thrombus. In cases where the color flow is not seen on color Doppler or spectral Doppler, it is a good practice to assess the vein with power Doppler as the latter is most sensitive to flow

COMPETENT SAPHENOFEMORAL JUNCTION

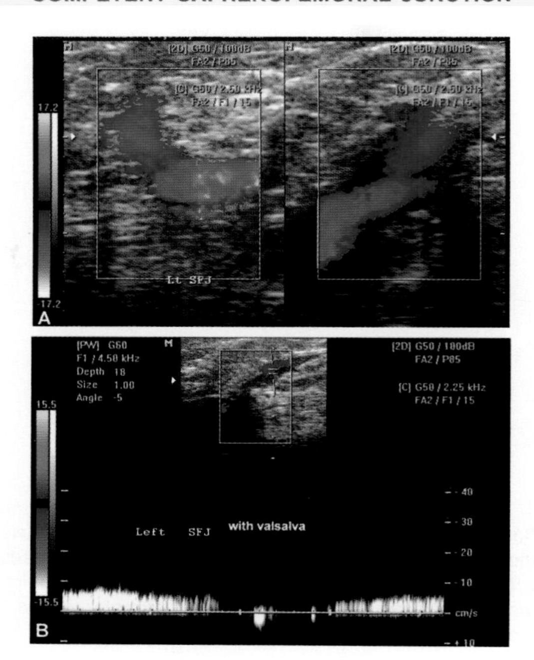

FIGURES 10.7A and B

(A) Color Doppler image shows similar color code in both common femoral and great saphenous vein due to similar direction of blood flow in both veins, (B) Duplex Doppler shows normal monophasic flow on the left side of trace with complete cessation of flow during Valsalva maneuver in middle part of trace followed by normal flow post-Valsalva suggestive of competent saphenofemoral junction

INCOMPETENT SAPHENOFEMORAL JUNCTION

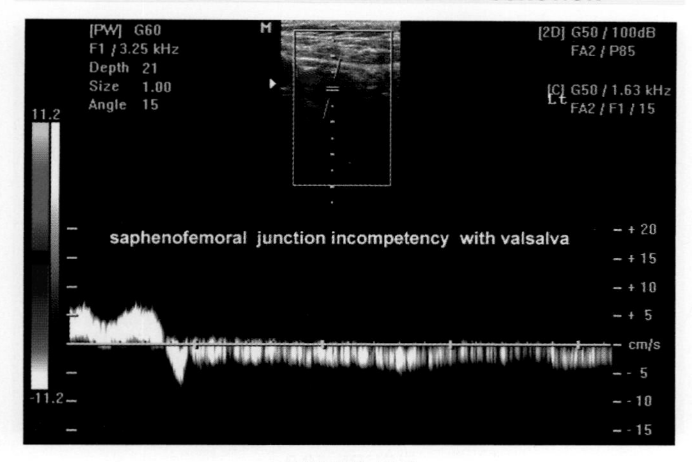

FIGURE 10.8

Duplex Doppler image through the saphenofemoral junction shows monophasic forward flow before Valsalva maneuver on the left side of trace with continuous reverse flow on the right side of the trace during Valsalva suggestive of incompetent saphenofemoral junction

THROMBUS AT SAPHENOFEMORAL JUNCTION

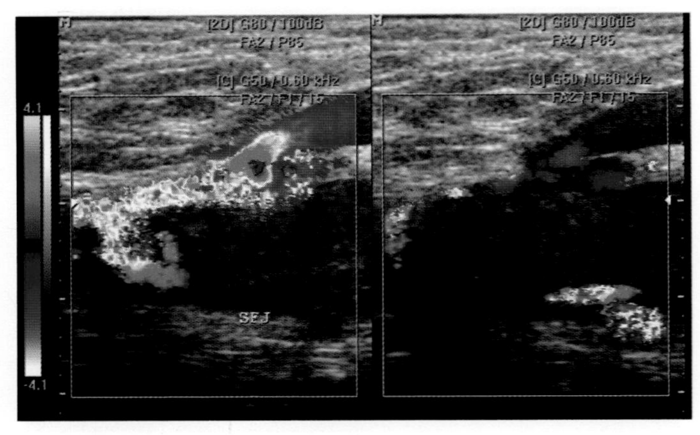

FIGURE 10.9

Color Doppler image at the level of saphenofemoral junction shows an intraluminal subacute hypoechoic thrombus in common femoral vein with partially patent saphenofemoral junction. The presence of multiple colors at the saphenofemoral junction indicates turbulence due to obstruction to the blood flow

During deep venous thrombosis (DVT) examination, the following should be checked:

1. Whether thrombosis present?
2. If yes, the extent and age of thrombosis
3. Whether the thrombosis is adherent to the vessel vessel wall and
4. The cause of thrombosis

During chronic venous insufficient (CVI), the following should be checked:

1. Whether insufficiency present?
2. If yes, the proximal and distil unit of insufficiency
3. Is the deep venous system patent and competent.

Specific problems and solutions

Poor visualization of the femoral vein in the adductor canal.
Support the thigh from behind with the left hand during the examination. Otherwise, try a posterior apporach for imaging the distal portions of the adductor canal.

The leg appears too swollen for ultrasound examination.
First consider alternative modalities. If this is not possible, locate the femoral vein in the groin and also locate the popliteal vein. Both sites can always be evaluated with ultrasound. The findings, though minimal, are useful for selecting therapeutic options when thrombosis is present.

Thrombosis is present, but the pelvic vessels are difficult to evaluate.
The external iliac vein can almost always be evaluated in its distal portion, but often the proximal end of the thrombus cannot be seen. There is usually no difficulty in compressing the vena cava. However, this finding is usually adequate if conservative treatment is desired, since ultrasound has demonstrated involvement at the pelvic level while excluding vena cava thrombosis.

Thrombosis is absent, but the pelvic vessels are difficult to evaluate.
If there is no reason to suspect that isolated pelvic vein thrombosis is present (e.g., pelvic mass, malignant lymphoma), thrombosis at that level can be indirectly excluded by a normal response of the common femoral vein to a Valsalva maneuver.

Significant atherosclerosis of the accompanying arteries creates acoustic shadows that obscure the veins.
Try changing the transducer position to scan past the artery and interrogate the vein directly.

The veins in the lower leg cannot be positively identified.
In a patient with a very thick calf, adjust the transducer position to minimize the distance from the transducer face to the veins of interest. If they still cannot be adequately visualized, try flexing the leg over the edge of the table.

Findings and pitfalls

Echogenic lumen (suspected thrombosis)
Intravascular echoes can be caused by overamplification of the B-mode image (B-mode gain too high) or unfavorable acoustic conditions.

Echo-free lumen (no sign of thrombosis)
Fresh thrombi may appear sonolucent

No detectable flow signal in the vessel lumen (suspected thrombosis)
Very slow flow may be below the threshold of detection even with optimum instrument settings. Often, a color signal cannot be obtained just proximal or distal to thrombosis, in the lower leg, or in a standing examination. Shadowing from calcified plaque in the accompanying artery can prevent color flow imaging.

Detectable flow signal in the vessel lumen (no sign of thrombosis)
Thrombosis that is incomplete or partially recanalized may produce a detectable flow signal, so make certain that color fills the lumen before excluding thrombosis. Occasionally, this is difficult to achieve even in healthy subjects, which is why distal compression is often used. This technique may cause a partial thrombosis to become swamped with echoes.

Chapter Eleven

Intravascular Ultrasound (IVUS)

NORMAL APPEARANCE

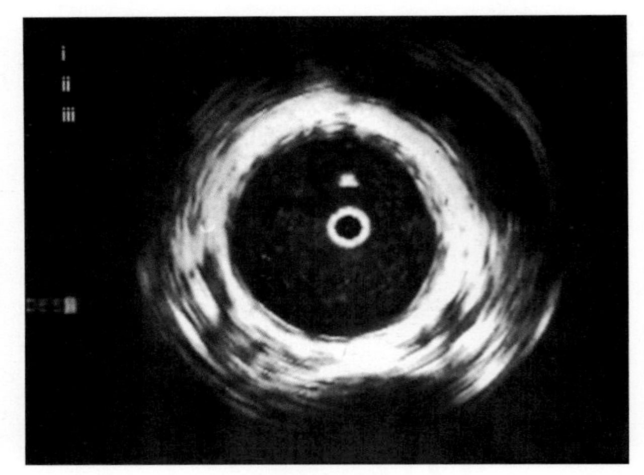

FIGURE 11.1

IVUS image in a normal subject: 3-layered appearance:

(i) Thin inner echogenic layer (internal elastic lamina)
(ii) Middle hypoechoic layer (media)
(iii) Outermost echogenic layer (adventitia). Blood around catheter seen as speckled pattern

INTIMAL HYPERPLASIA

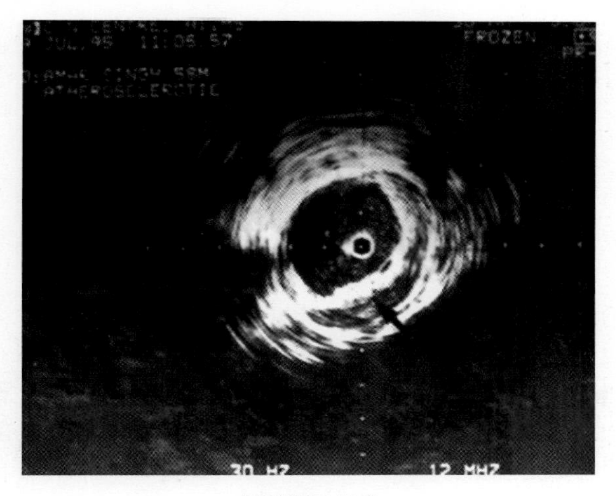

FIGURE 11.2

IVUS image showing eccentric increase in thickness of inner layer (arrow) suggestive of intimal hyperplasia

FIBROUS PLAQUE

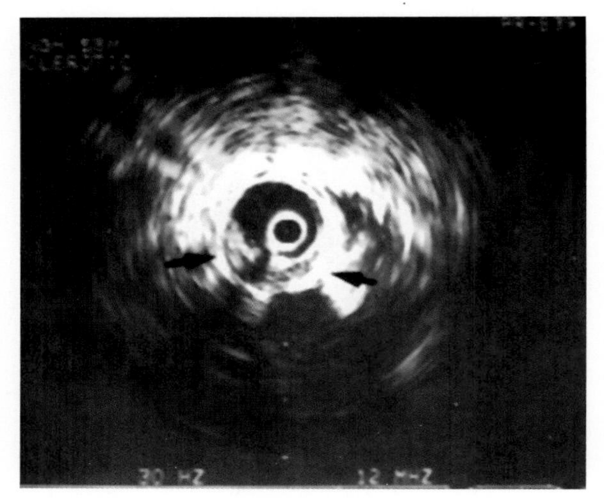

FIGURE 11.3

IVUS image shows fibrous plaque (arrow) with outer echogenic line with distal acoustic shadowing (calcium)

PLAQUE

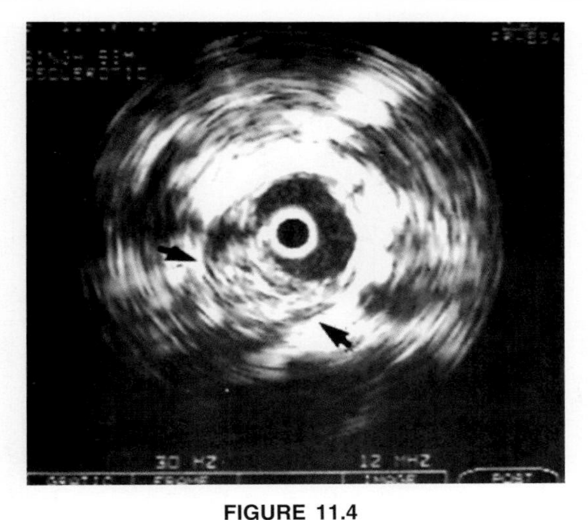

FIGURE 11.4

IVUS image of aorta shows mixed echogenicity plaque (arrows)

AORTOARTERITIS

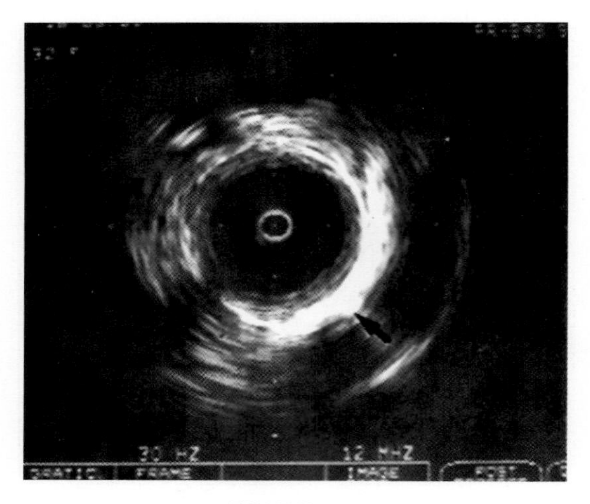

FIGURE 11.5

IVUS image shows thick echogenic media and adventitia (arrow) with thin innermost layer, suggesting aortoarteritis

RENAL ARTERY STENOSIS

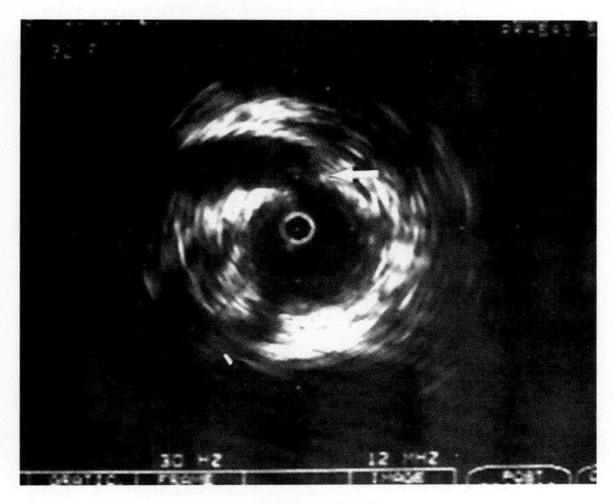

FIGURE 11.6

IVUS image shows renal artery take-off (arrow) seen in upper part of image with stenosis at its ostium. Aortic wall shows thick echogenic media suggestive of renal artery stenosis secondary to aortoarteritis

Chapter Twelve

Doppler in Gynecology

UTERINE ARTERY WAVEFORM

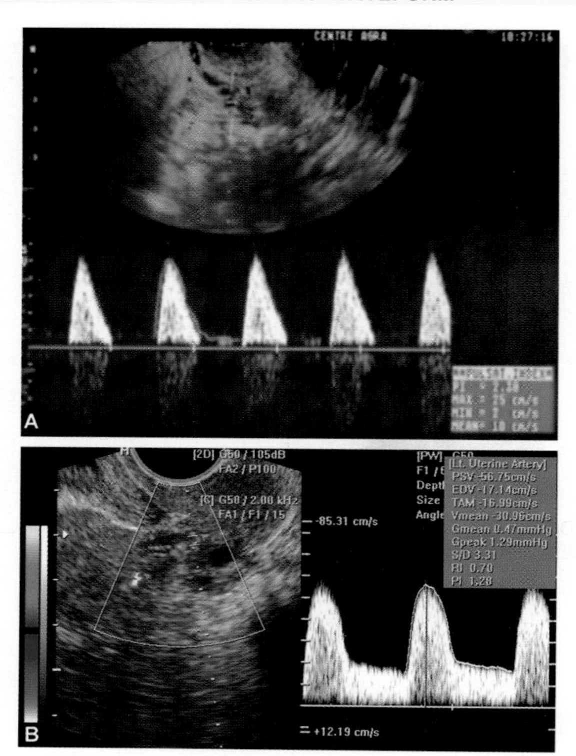

FIGURES 12.1A and B

(A) During the early proliferative phase shows predominantly systolic flow with minimal or no diastolic flow, (B) At 10th of menstrual cycle showing low impedance flow with significant forward diastolic flow with moderate RI values

UTERINE VASCULATURE

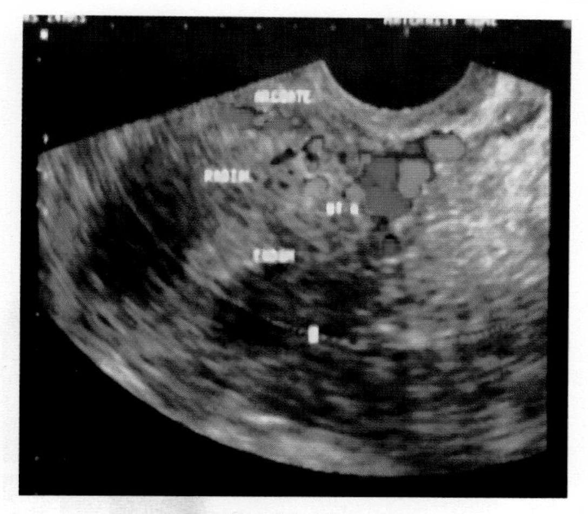

FIGURE 12.2

Color Doppler showing the pattern of uterine vasculature, i.e. uterine, arcuate and radial arteries

OVARIAN VASCULARITY

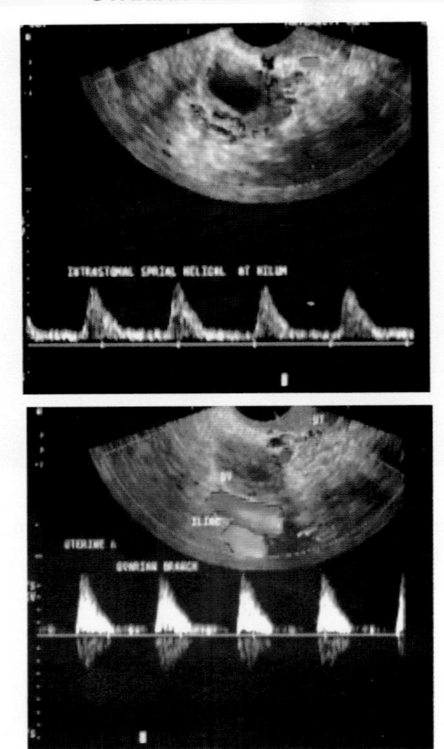

FIGURES 12.3A and B

(A) Ovarian arterial flow pattern. Intrastromal color flow is also noted,
(B) Ovarian branch of uterine artery

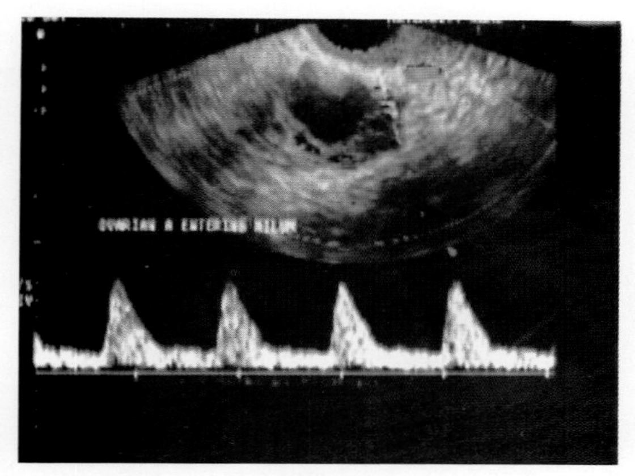

FIGURE 12.3C

Spectral waveform of the ovarian artery high systolic and forward low diastolic flow

CORPUS LUTEUM CYST

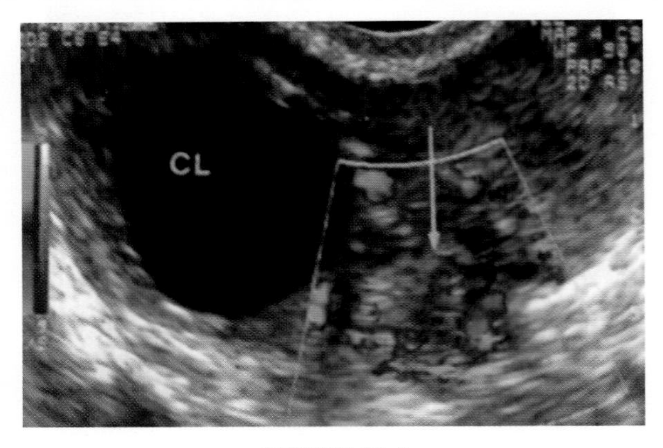

FIGURE 12.4

Color flow pattern of the corpus luteum—mild peripheral vascularity is noted. On duplex Doppler, low impedance flow is characteristic

COLOR DOPPLER IMAGE FIBROID

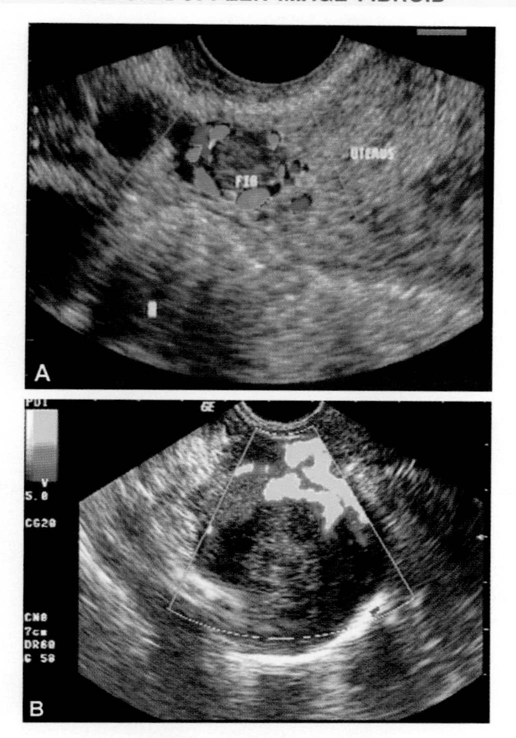

FIGURES 12.5A and B

Color doppler image fibroid (A) and power Doppler image (B) demonstrates peripheral vascularity in a fibroid which is characteristically of high impedance pattern. Infrequently central stromal vascularity may also be noted especially in cases of red degeneration during pregnancy or presence of concomitant adenomyomatous tissue

ECTOPIC PREGNANCY

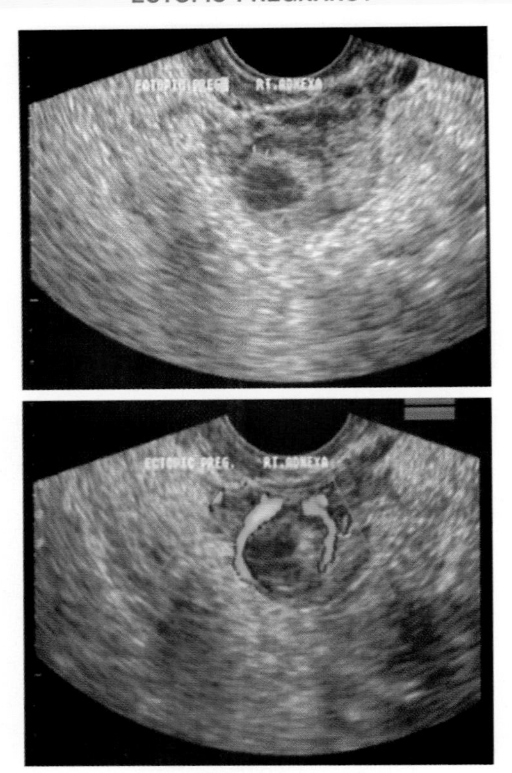

FIGURES 12.6A and B

(A) Gray scale image showing a complex right adnexal mass (B) Color Doppler image shows peripheral vascularity around the mass creating a “ring of fire” appearance

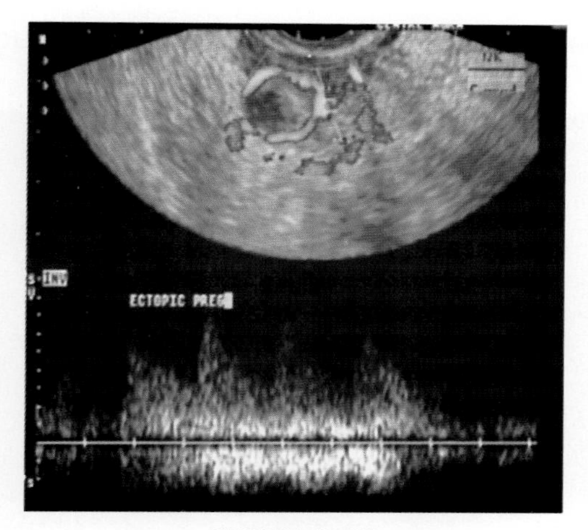

FIGURE 12.6C

Duplex Doppler demonstrates trophoblastic flow pattern with high PSV and EDV and low RI and PI values

FERTILE ENDOMETRIUM AND FUNCTIONAL FOLLICLE

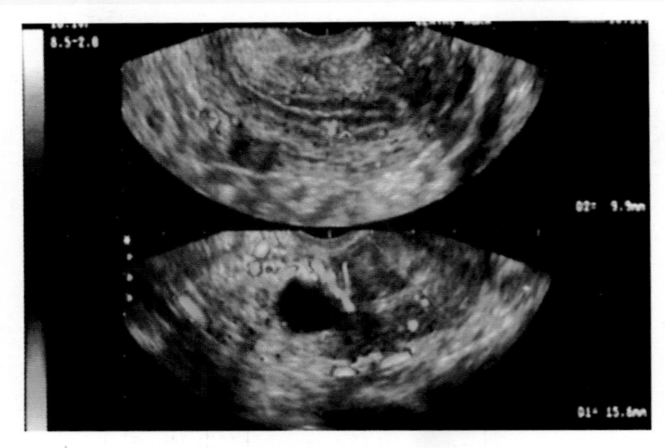

FIGURE 12.7

Color Doppler image shows ring of angiogenesis around the dominant follicle of the ovary suggestive of functional follicle (bottom). Vascularity is also seen in the endometrium suggestive of fertile endometrium (top)

POLYCYSTIC OVARIAN DISEASE (PCOD)

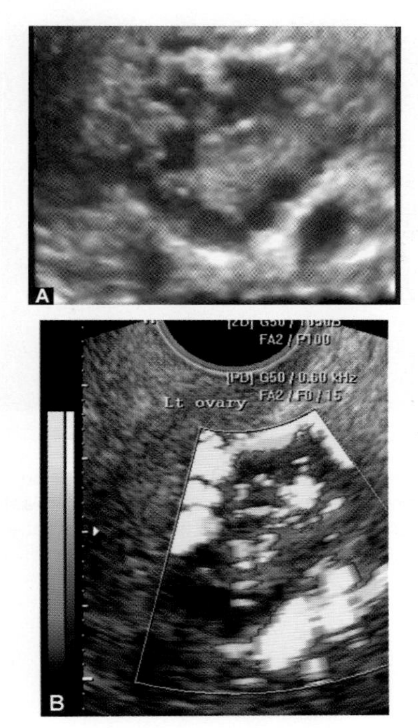

FIGURES 12.8A and B

(A) 3D Gray scale image showing an enlarged ovary with multiple small follicles arranged at the periphery of the ovary associated with increased stromal echogenicity, (B) Color Doppler image shows high intrastromal vascularity suggestive of angiogenic stroma which is characteristic of PCOD

OVARIAN STIMULATION

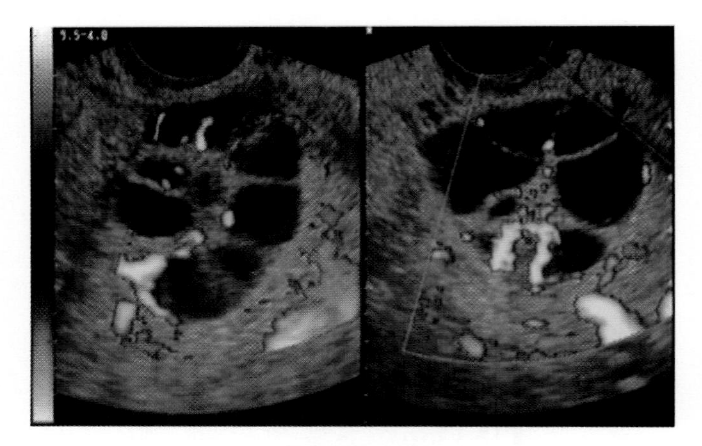

FIGURE 12.9

Color Doppler image shows high intraovarian perfusion seen in a case of ovarian stimulation suggestive of increased vascularity in response to the stimulus

SONOSALPINGOGRAPHY

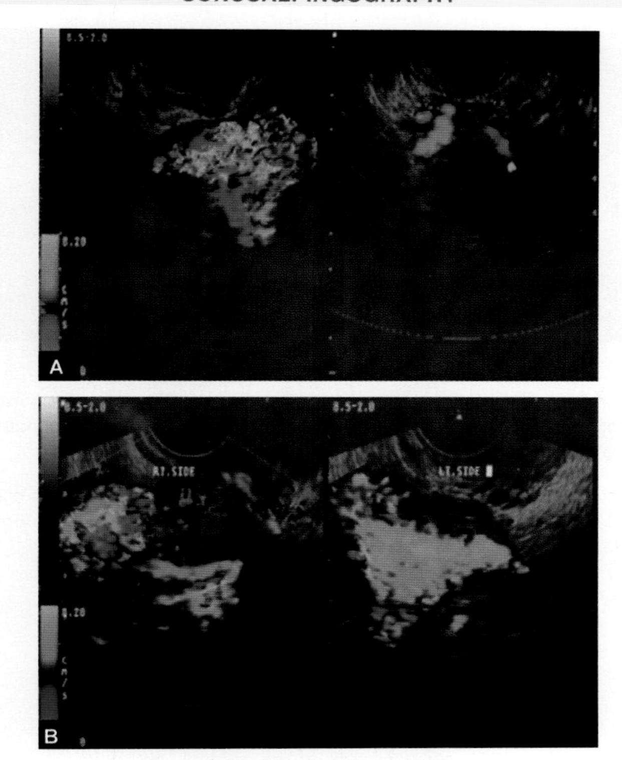

FIGURES 12.10A and B

Color Doppler image shows color spill from the fimbrial end on both sides arising due to spillage of saline / contrast from the fimbrial end into the peritoneal cavity confirming the tubal patency. But partial obstruction or deformed fimbrae cannot be ruled out

ENDOMETRIAL POLYP

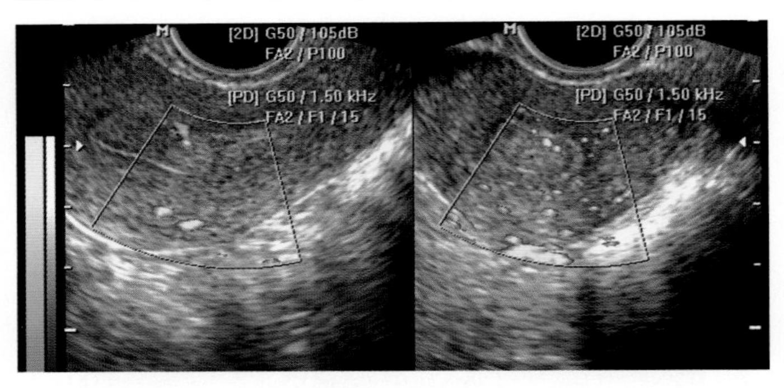

FIGURE 12.11

Color Doppler image shows fine vascularity within a well-defined echogenic mass within the endometrium suggestive of an endometrial polyp. Absence of flow will be seen in cases of blood clot

ENDOMETRIAL CARCINOMA

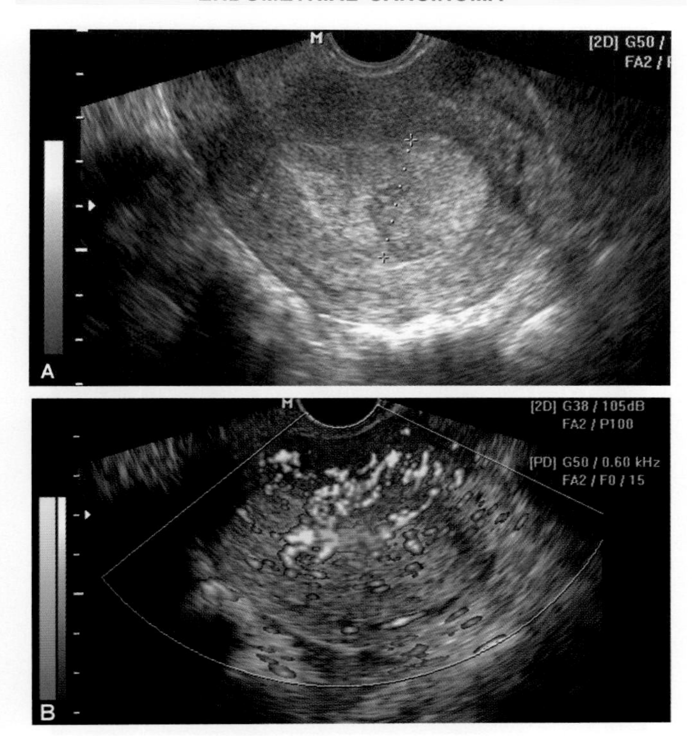

FIGURES 12.12A and B

(A) Gray scale image shows endometrial carcinoma presenting as increased endometrial thickening, (B) Power Doppler image shows high and haphazard vascularity within the endometrium suggestive of malignant lesion, i.e. endometrial carcinoma

CERVICAL CARCINOMA

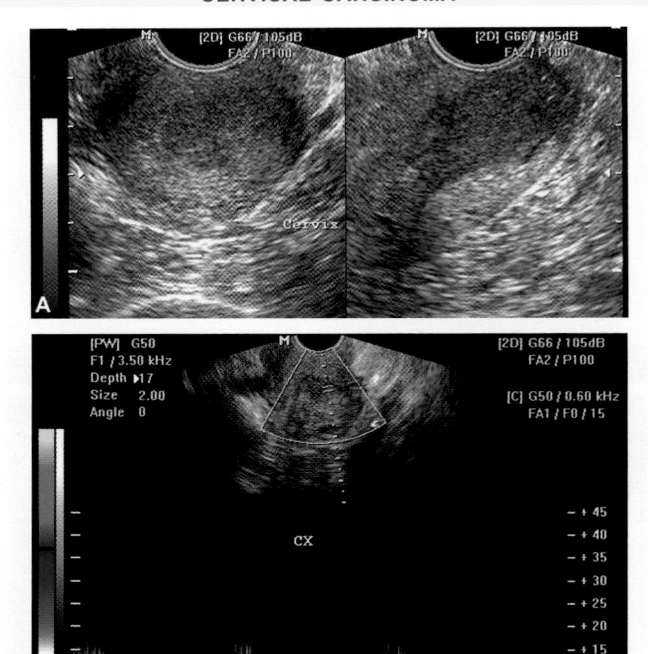

FIGURES 12.13A and B

(A) Gray scale image shows hypoechoic mass in cervix, (B) Color Doppler image shows vascularity in cervical mass with low resistance flow suggestive of malignant etiology

ENDOMETRIAL VASCULARITY

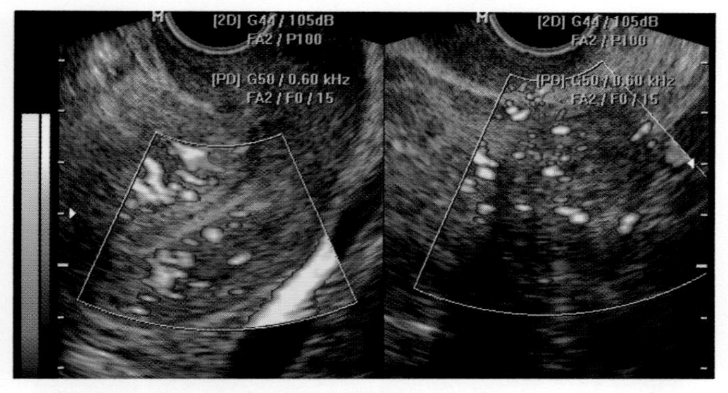

FIGURE 12.14

Power Doppler image shows vascularity reaching up to the endometrial lining. This pattern should always be assessed while examining the patients of infertility or those undergoing embryo transfers into the endometrial cavity

ENDOMETRIOMA OF OVARY

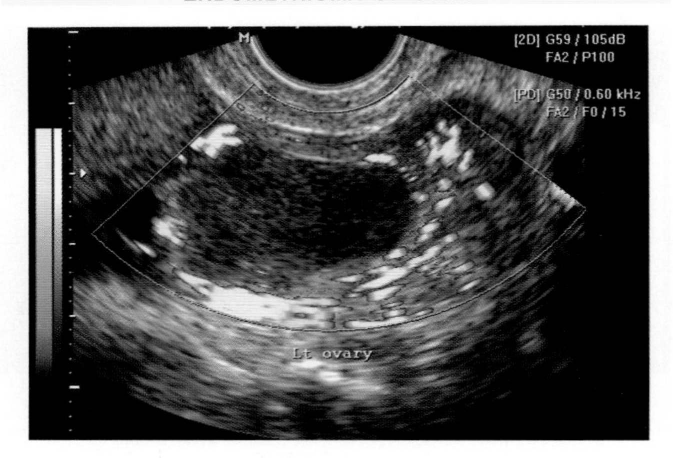

FIGURE 12.15

Power Doppler demonstrates peripheral vascularity in an endometrioma of ovary. On duplex Doppler, the flow pattern will be of high resistance pattern differentiating it from corpus luteum

UTERINE ARTERIOVENOUS MALFORMATION

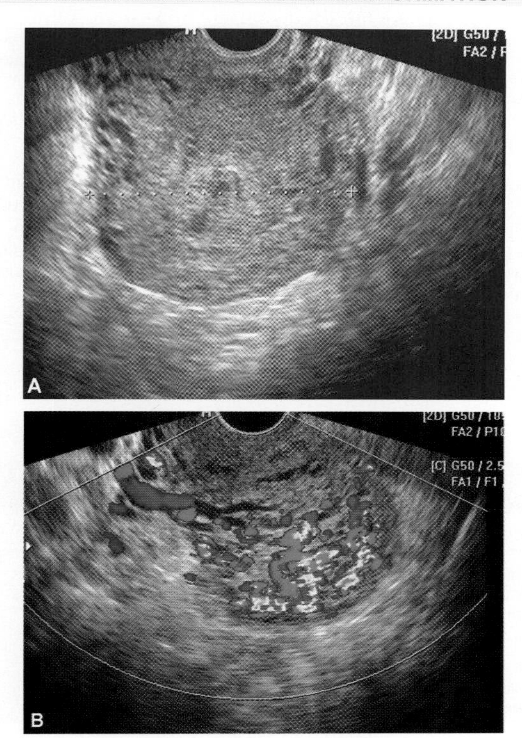

FIGURES 12.16A and B

(A) Gray scale image shows heteroechoic mass within in the bulky uterus with few cystic areas, (B) Color Doppler shows extensive network of the vessels within the uterine myometrium reaching up to the mass

Classification of ovarian masses using B-mode ultrasound

Mass	Fluid		Inner margin		Interpretation
Unilocular	Clear	(0)	Smooth	(0)	
	Internal echoes	(1)	Irregular	(2)	
Multilocular	Clear	(1)	Smooth	(1)	
	Internal echoes	(1)	Irregular	(2)	
Cystic-Solid	Clear	(1)	Smooth	(1)	
	Internal echoes	(2)	Irregular	(2)	Ultrasound score
					<2 Benign
Papillary growths	Suspicious	(1)	Definitive	(2)	3-4 Equivocal
Solid area	Homogeneous	(1)	Echogenic	(2)	>4 Suspicious
Peritonial fluid	Not present	(0)	Present	(1)	
Unilateral/bilateral	Unilateral	(0)	Bilateral	(1)	

Color duplex classification of ovarian masses

Color Doppler		Resistance index		Interpretation
–No detectable vessels	(0)		(0)	
–Uniform seperate vessels	(1)	>0.40	(1)	Color Doppler score
–Random vascular	(2)	<0.40	(2)	<2 Benign
				3-4 Suspicious
If corpus luteum is suspected: Repeat ultrasound in the proliferative phase of the next menstrual cycle				

Chapter Thirteen

Doppler in Obstetrics

EARLY PREGNANCY

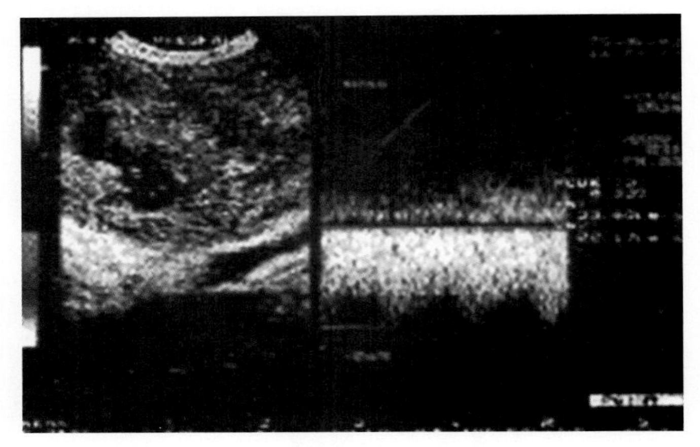

FIGURE 13.1

Trophoblastic flow detected in early pregnancy reveals low impedance pattern characterized by low RI and PI values for maximum vascular flow to the developing embryo

EARLY PREGNANCY

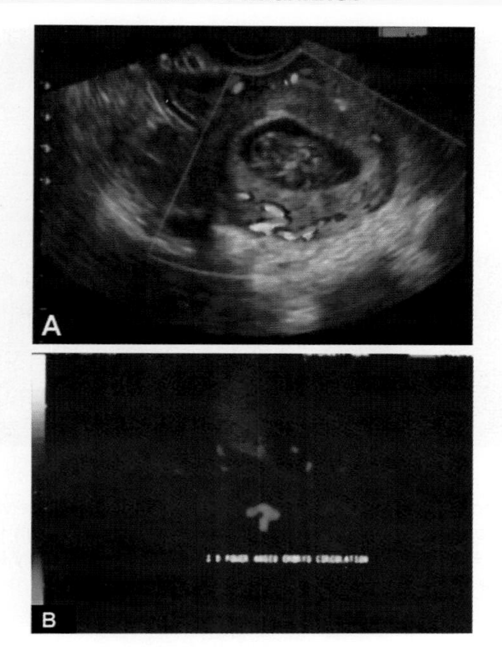

FIGURES 13.2A and B

(A) Color Doppler at nine weeks of gestation shows the presence of color flow in the heart and aorta and cranial cavity. Color Doppler is very useful to visualize the beating heart, if there is any confusion regarding the presence or absence of cardiac activity in early pregnancy, (B) 3D power angiogram showing early embryonic circulation. As power Doppler is more sensitive than color Doppler, PDI is useful in assessing the viability of fetus early in pregnancy

PREGNANCY-7 WEEKS

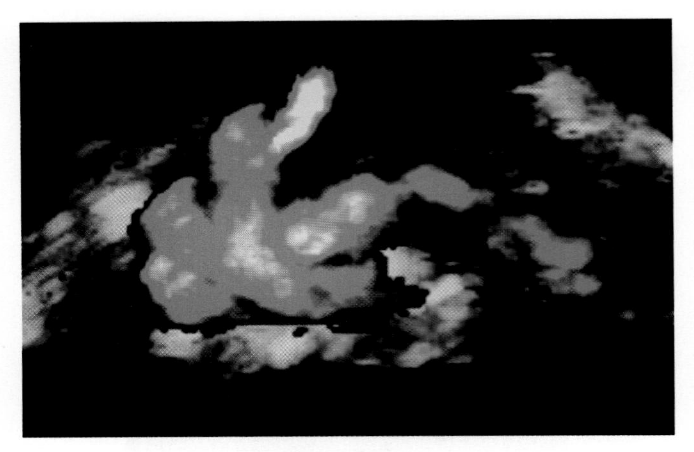

FIGURE 13.3

Power Doppler image at 7 weeks shows two arteries and one vein in the umbilical cord. As two-vessel cord is associated with a high incidence of congenital anomalies, PDI can be used in early pregnancy to assess the number of vessels in umbilical cord

THREE-VESSEL CORD

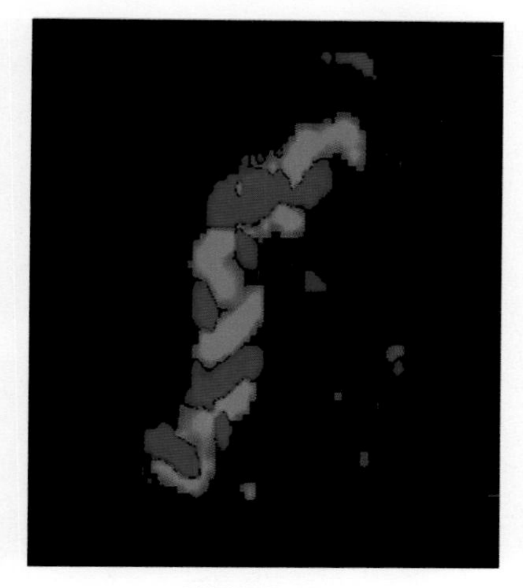

FIGURE 13.4

3D angiographic image shows a three vessel cord. Such images can be used to assess the coiling index of umbilical cord. As uncoiled or hypo-coiled cords are related with congenital anomalies, 3D angiographic image of umbilical cord assumes significance

UTERINE ARTERY FLOW—NON PREGNANT STATE

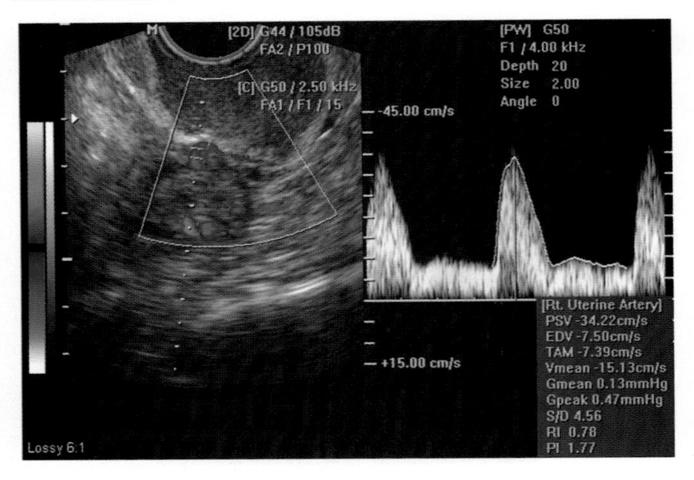

FIGURE 13.5

Flow pattern of uterine artery in nonpregnant state shows high systolic flow and low diastolic flow. This pattern is usually seen in the post-ovulatory phase of menstrual cycle. The diastolic flow is much less or even absent in early phase of menstrual cycle

UTERINE ARTERY FLOW IN PREGNANCY

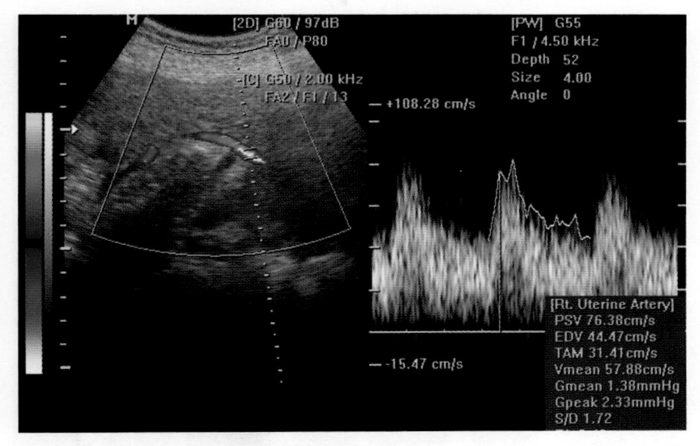

FIGURE 13.6

Flow pattern of uterine artery in pregnancy shows high velocity flow during both systolic and diastolic phase with multiple peaks through diastole suggesting turbulence of flow subsequent to the increased demand of blood in pregnant state

PREGNANCY-BEFORE 24 WEEKS

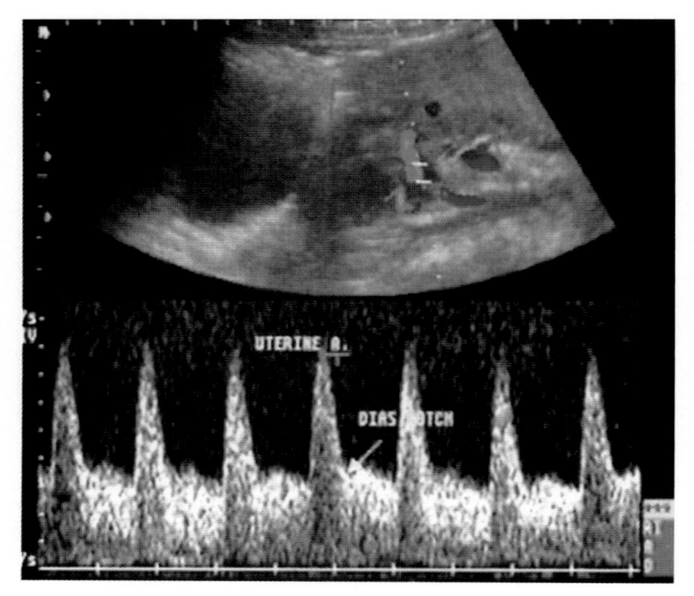

FIGURE 13.7

Uterine artery flow pattern before 24 weeks of gestation shows a diastolic notch between the systolic and diastolic flow. The importance of this notch lies in the fact that it is present up to 24-26 weeks of gestation. If persistence after 26 weeks of gestation is indicative of uterine insufficiency that may lead to fetal vascular compromise

PREGNANCY 24-26 WEEKS

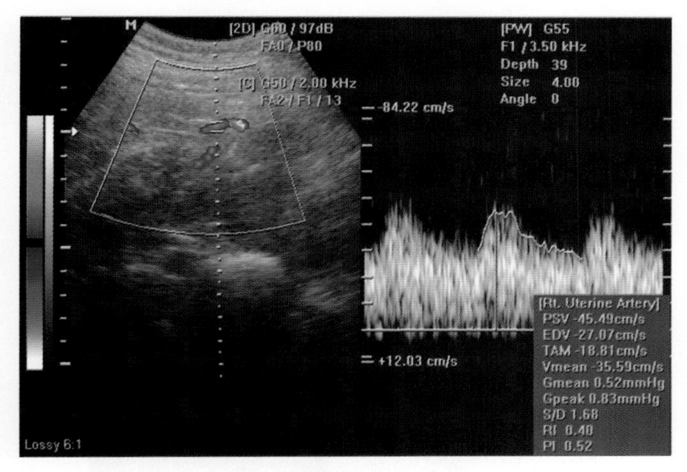

FIGURE 13.8

Uterine artery flow showing complete disappearance of the diastolic notch by 24-26 weeks of gestation suggestive of good uterine vascular flow

INCOMPLETE ABORTION

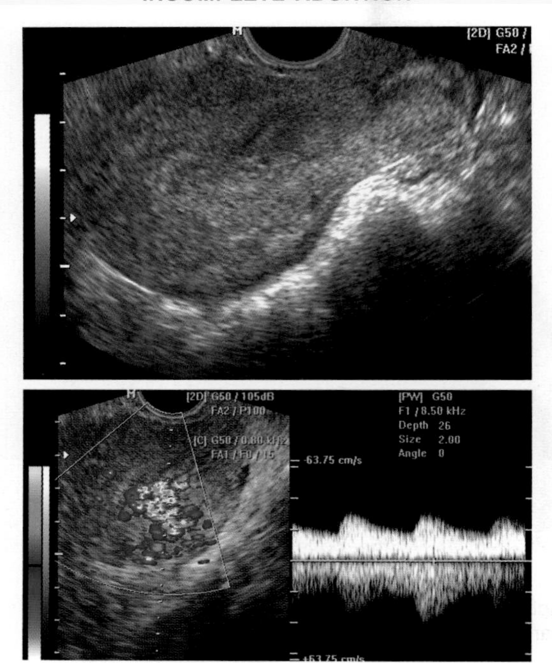

FIGURES 13.9A and B

(A) Gray scale image showing a bulky uterus with echogenicity at 3rd postabortal week indicating possible incomplete abortion, (B) Color Doppler showing high vascularity in the region of increased echogenicity with low resistance flow (indicated by significant diastolic flow) confirming incomplete abortion. Any persistence of low resistance flow after 2 weeks of abortion is highly suggestive of incomplete abortion or retained products of conceptus

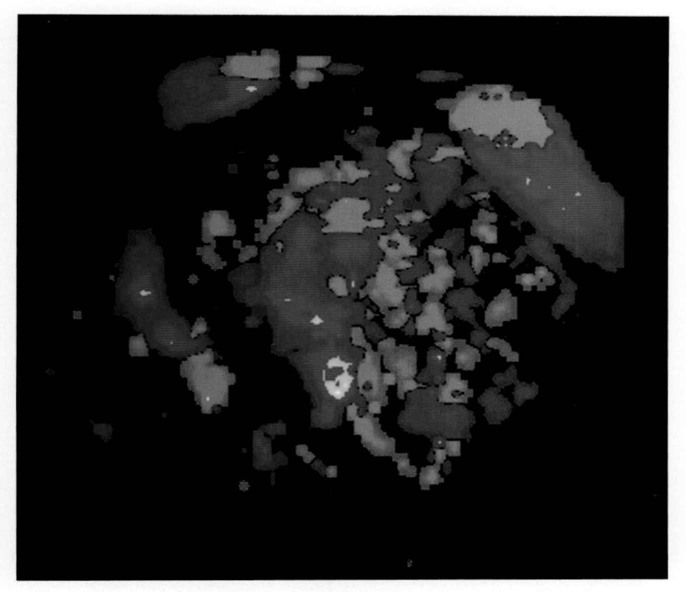

FIGURE 13.9C

3D angiographic image shows the haphazard arrangement of the vascular channels associated with incomplete abortion

UMBILICAL FLOW PATTERN-NORMAL

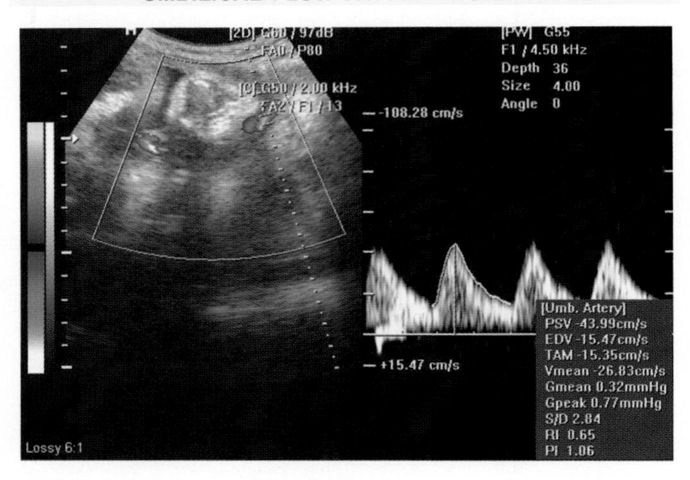

FIGURE 13.10

Normal umbilical artery flow pattern reveals a low resistance flow. Under normal conditions, the umbilical artery reveals RI values of less than 0.7 and SD ratio of less than 3 after 24-26 weeks of gestation

PLACENTAL INSUFFICIENCY

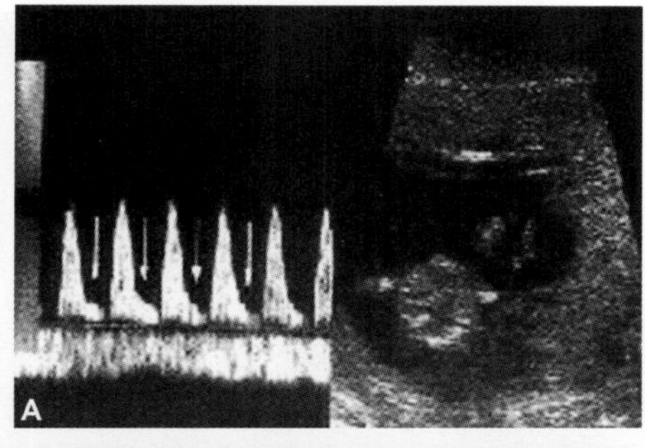

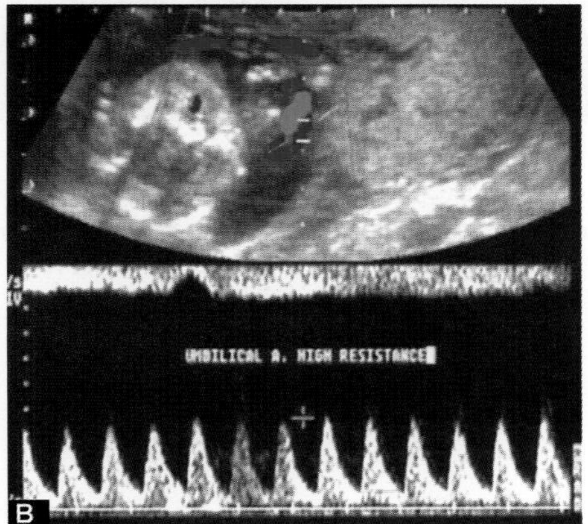

FIGURES 13.11A and B

(A) Doppler at 30 weeks of gestation shows reduced diastolic flow in the umbilical artery signifying placental insufficiency, (B) RI in umbilical artery is more than 0.7 indicating decreased diastolic flow

IUGR

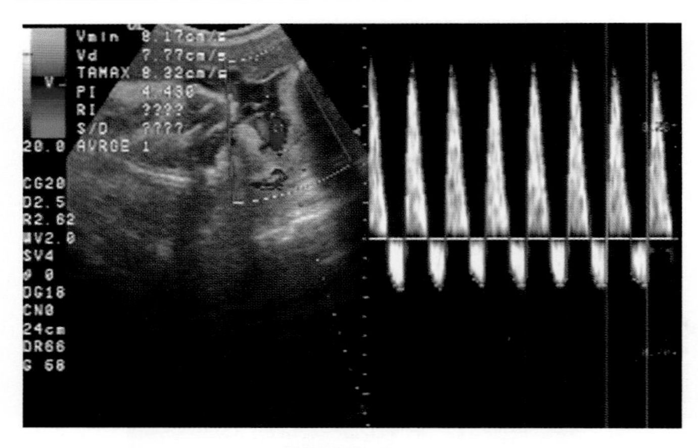

FIGURE 13.12

Umbilical artery waveform in a case of IUGR shows reversal of diastolic flow signifying impending fetal death. Umbilical artery waveform normally reveals good forward diastolic flow; hence absence or reverse diastolic flow is abnormal

UMBILICAL VEIN-NORMAL FLOW PATTERN

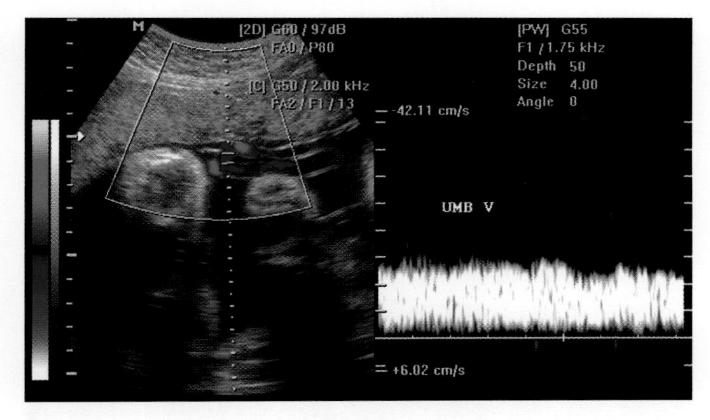

FIGURE 13.13

Duplex Doppler shows normal flow pattern in umbilical vein with continuous flow with respiratory variations

FETAL AORTA-FLOW PATTERN

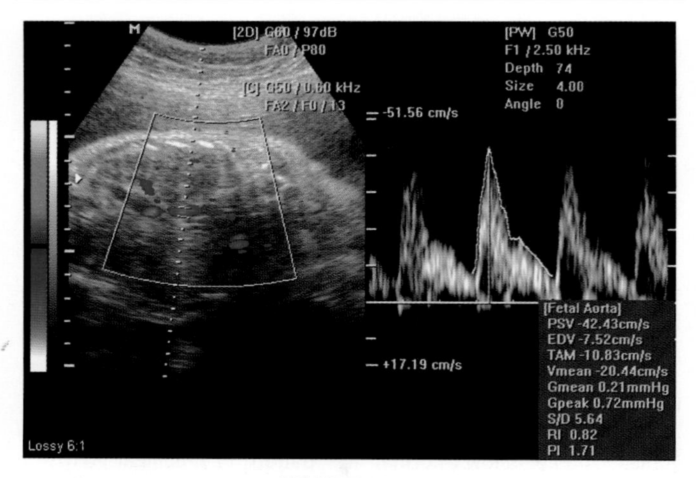

FIGURE 13.14

Normal flow pattern in fetal aorta shows high systolic and low diastolic flow. The RI values of more than 0.9 and PI values of more than 2.5 should be taken as abnormal indicating fetal hypoxia

IUGR-FLOW PATTERN IN AORTA

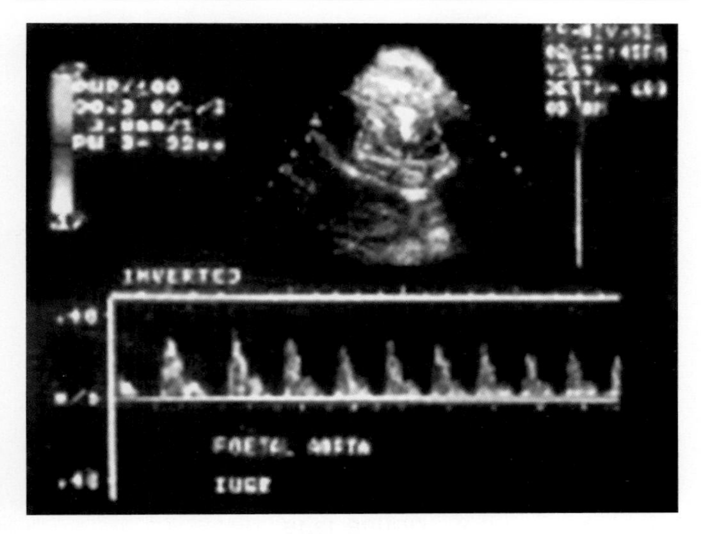

FIGURE 13.15

Flow pattern of aorta in IUGR showing complete loss of flow during the late phase of diastole suggestive of high peripheral resistance indicating fetal hypoxia and IUGR

CIRCLE OF WILLIS

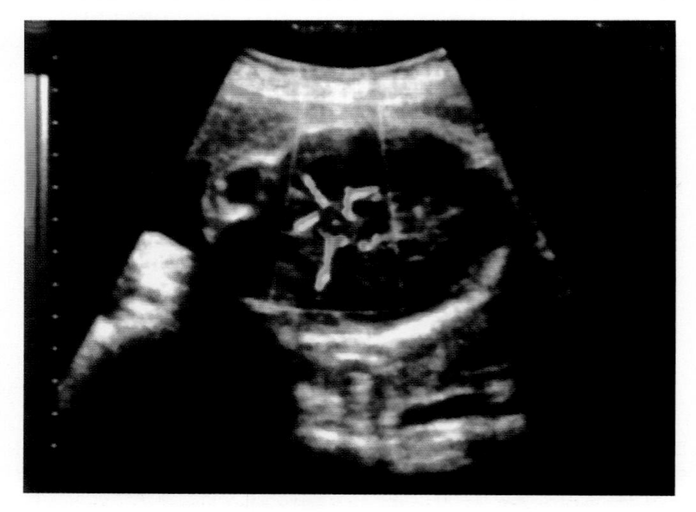

FIGURE 13.16

Doppler image of the fetal circle of Willis shows the bilateral middle cerebral, anterior cerebral and posterior communicating arteries. This image to used to get the flow pattern from fetal MCA

FETAL MIDDLE CEREBRAL ARTERY

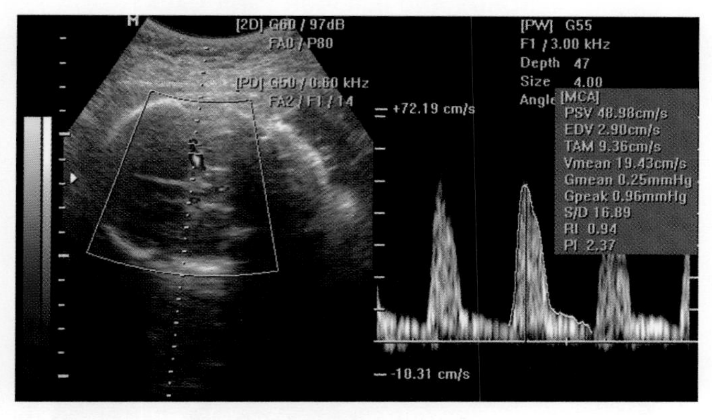

FIGURE 13.17

Duplex Doppler shows normal pattern of flow in fetal middle cerebral artery with high systolic flow and low forward diastolic flow. Absence or reverse diastolic flow is abnormal. If the RI value of fetal MCA is constantly below 0.7, then it is suggestive of cerebral vasodilatation secondary to fetal hypoxia

FLOW PATTERN IN DUCTUS VENOSUS AND INFERIOR VENA CAVA

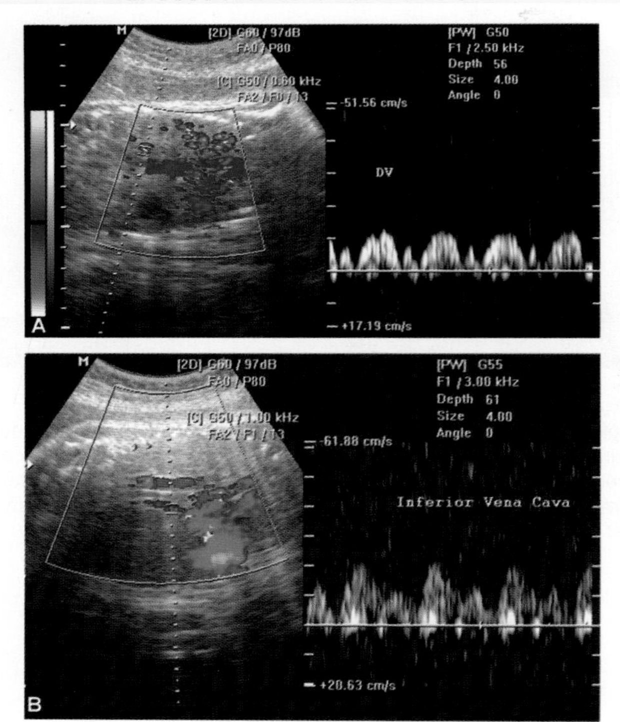

FIGURES 13.18A and B

(A) Duplex Doppler showing normal pulsatile flow in ductus venosus with 3-wave pattern and no or minimal reverse component, (B) Duplex Doppler showing normal pulsatile flow in inferior vena cava similar to that seen in the ductus venosus

FETAL HYPOXIA

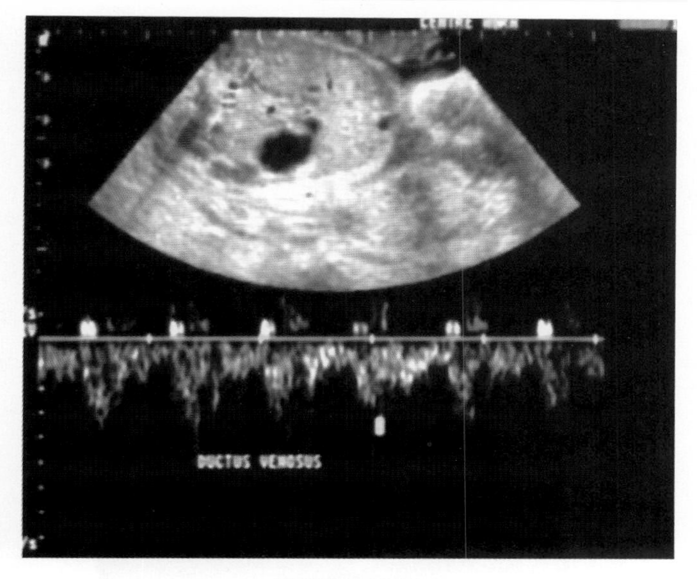

FIGURE 13.19

Duplex Doppler image showing an increased reversed flow in ductus venosus indicative of fetal hypoxia and acidosis

HYDATIDIFORM MOLE

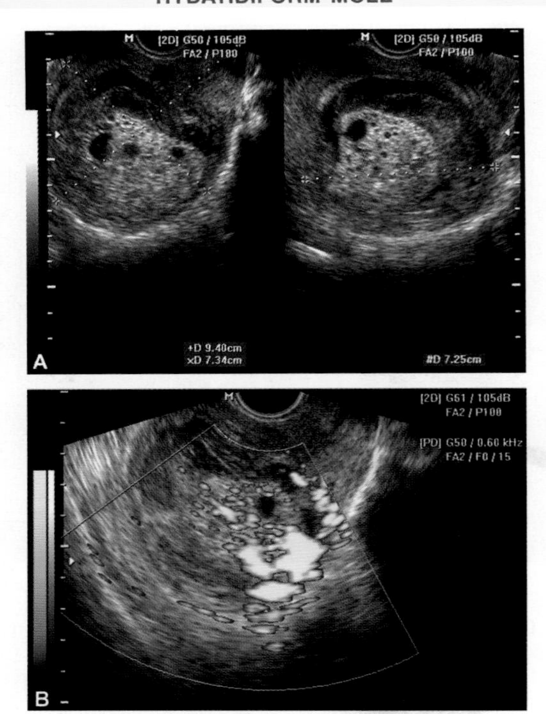

FIGURES 13.20A and B

(A) Gray scale image shows a predominantly echogenic mass with multiple cystic areas of varying sizes in a bulky uterus with history of amenorrhea suggestive of hydatiform mole, (B) Power Doppler image shows high vascularity around the lesion indicative of trophoblastic pattern, thus confirming the diagnosis of hydatiform mole

CHORIOCARCINOMA

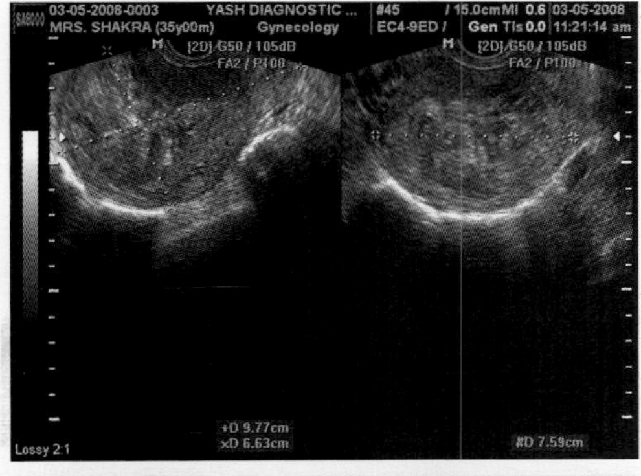

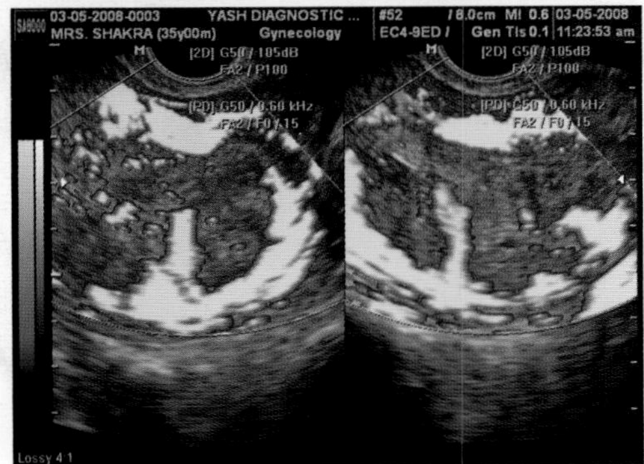

FIGURES 13.21A and B

(A) Gray scale image shows a heteroechoic mass in a bulky uterus with a history of recent abortion, (B) Power Doppler image shows high peripheral and central vascularity within the mass

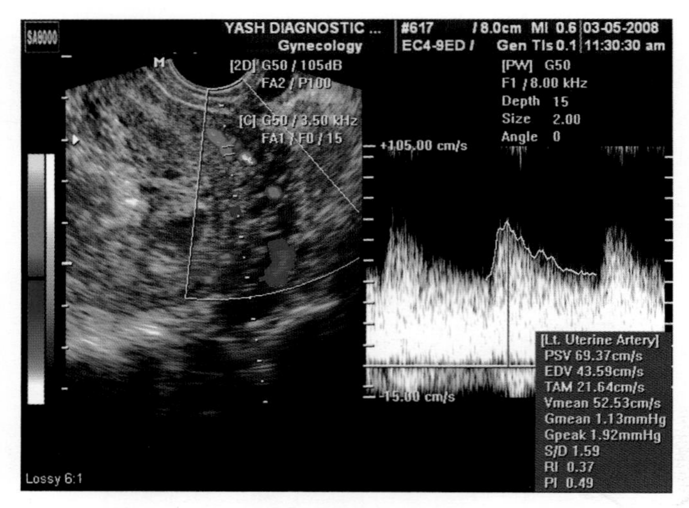

FIGURE 13.21C

Duplex Doppler shows uterine arterial flow resembling pregnancy with high PSV and low RI and PI values suggestive of presence of trophoblastic tissue

Absence of diastolic flow and reserve flow in the umbilical artery		
Effect on perinatal outcome	*Mean value*	*Range*
Mortality (%)	45	17-100
Gestational age (weeks)	31.6	29-33
Birthweight (g)	1056	910-1481
SGA (%)	68	53-100
Cesarean section due to fetal distress (%)	73	24-100
Apgar score <7 after 5 min (%)	26	7-69
Transfer to neonatal ICU (%)	84	77-97
Congenital anomalies (%)	10	0-24
Aneuploidy (%)	6.4	0-18

Blood Flow calsses in Spectral Patterns in Obstetrics Ultrasound

Class 0	PI < + 2 SD and continuous forward diastolic flow
Class I	PI ≥ + 2 SD and continuous forward flow
Class II	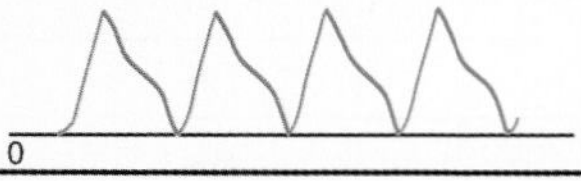 0
Class IIIa	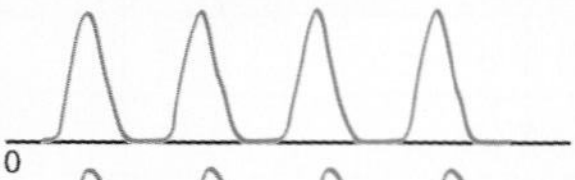 0
Class IIIb	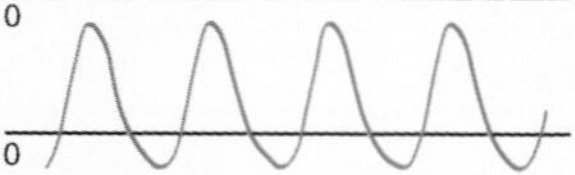 0

Normal values in the fetal aorta		
Peak systolic velocity	*Mean value*	*Range*
V max	m	m + 2 SD
25 weeks' gestation	80 cm/s	65-95 cm/s
37 weeks' gestation	100 cm/s	80-130 cm/s
>39 weeks' gestation	90 cm/s	70-115 cm/s

INDEX

A

B

C

D

L

M

N

O

P

Q

R

S

T

U

V

W

Z